A Guide to...
Basic Health & Disease in Birds

Their Management, Care & Well-being

Revised Edition

By Dr Michael J Cannon BVSc, MACVSc, GradDipEd.

I dedicate this revised edition to my wife, Marlene, for her support that is always there.

Published and Edited by ABK Publications ©

© **ABK Publications 2002**

First Published 1996 by
Australian Birdkeeper
PO Box 6288,
South Tweed Heads,
NSW. 2486. Australia.
Revised Edition 2002

ISBN 0 9577024 5 0

Disclaimer.
Very few drugs are registered for use in birds, and most usages and dose rates have been
extrapolated from mammalian therapeutics. Everyone using medications should be aware
that manufacturers of these drugs will not accept any responsibility for the 'off-label' use of
their drugs. The following dose rates and information are based on clinical trials and
practical experience, but unrecorded adverse side-effects may occur. Where possible, the
author has provided brand names for the drugs mentioned. These should not be taken as a
recommendation for one particular brand over another; but rather as a starting point for you
to find the drug of your choice. In most instances, contra indications (C/I) and side-effects are
not listed. This should not be taken to mean that there are none – many of these drugs have
not been used extensively, and reports on contra indications and side-effects are not
recorded at date of publication.

Front Cover:
Top left: Blue & Gold Macaw
Centre left: Scaly-face Mite in Budgerigar causing deformed beak
(Photograph Michael J Cannon)
Bottom left: Blue-faced Parrot Finch
Bottom right: Sulphur-crested Cockatoo with PBFD
(Photograph Stuart Horton)
Back Cover: Eastern Rosella cock

All cover photographs by ABK Publications except where indicated

All other photgraphs by Dr Michael J Cannon except where indicated.

Table of Contents

ABOUT THE AUTHOR

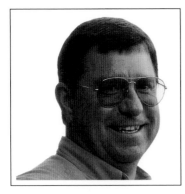

Michael J Cannon
BVSc, MACVSc (Avian Health), GradDipEd.

Graduated from University of Sydney in 1976.
Private practice in Forestville until 1979, then moved
to private practice in Wollongong until present.
MACVSc by examination in Avian Health in 1985.
President – Avicultural Society of NSW 1989 – 1991
Chairman – Research and Development
Subcommittee of Avicultural Federation and
Development Subcommittee of Avicultural Federation of Australia since 1986.

Developed and maintained an interest in avian medicine and surgery since
graduation. Maintains a small collection of Australian Parrots and is involved in
rehabilitation of Australian native animals, particularly birds.

Teacher-in-charge Zookeeping – Sydney Institute of Technology 1990 – 2001.

President Australian Branch, Association of Avian Veterinarians 1992 – 1993.

President Avian Health Chapter, Australian College Veterinary Scientists 1992 –
2000.

Consultant Veterinarian to Australian Wildlife Park, Eastern Creek, since 1990.

Michael has been contributing to **Australian Birdkeeper Magazine** almost
since its inception. A dedicated and tireless worker for the cause of aviculture in
Australia, Michael has gained enormous respect from aviculturists and veterinarians
alike throughout the world.

ACKNOWLEDGEMENTS

Both author and publisher would like to thank the following contributors for their
assistance in the production of this title.

Dr. Danny Brown, Dr. Bob Doneley, Stuart Horton, Russell Kingston, Dr. Jim Gill,
Dr. Branson Ritchie and Sheryll Steele-Boyce.

PUBLISHER'S NOTE

Since its first publication in 1996, **A Guide to Basic Health and Disease in
Birds** has proven to be one of the most sought after and respected titles worldwide in
this generic range of avian publications.

It is a credit to the author Dr Mike Cannon. His devotion and concern for all aspects
of avian health and husbandry have again been reflected in this revised and updated
edition.

It is with pleasure and pride that **ABK Publications** avails to aviculturists of the
world this informative and valuable title.

Nigel Steele-Boyce

Why Do Birds Get Sick?

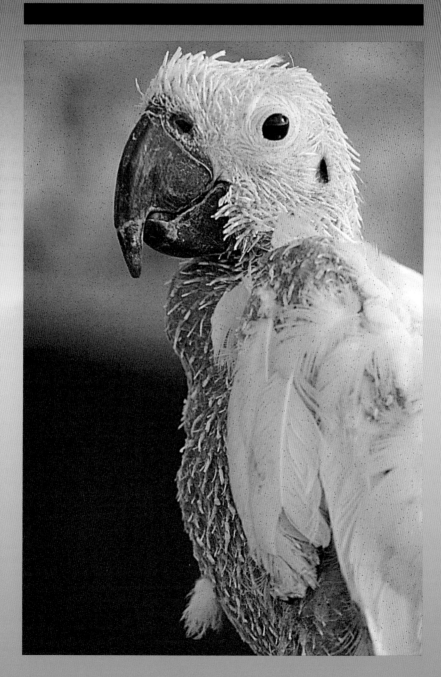

WHY DO BIRDS GET SICK?

People often ask me where a particular illness came from. It is not always possible to answer this other than in general terms. I feel that a little discussion on this theme may help you to understand the dynamics of disease.

Disease is caused by an interaction between the organism, the environment and the bird's health, or the strength of its immune system. We know that birds are constantly being exposed to organisms but do not develop illness. Why do some birds get sick and others remain healthy? It all depends on the dynamics affecting each of these three factors. You can have some influence on each factor.

The Organism

There are five basic disease organism groups:

1. Bacteria: Usually divided into Gram negative and Gram positive bacteria. Common examples are *E. coli*, *Staphylococcus* (Staphs), *Streptococcus* (Streps), *Salmonella*.
2. Fungi and yeasts: Common examples are ringworm, Megabacteria, *Aspergillus*.
3. Viruses: Common examples are Circovirus, Polyomavirus, Newcastle Disease, Pacheco's Virus.
4. Protozoan: Common examples are *Giardia*, *Toxoplasma*, *Coccisiosis* (*Eimeria*).
5. Parasites: Common examples are roundworm, *Capillaria*, tapeworm, lice, mites.

These organisms can build up in the environment. Every bird has an ability to fight them but will succumb if they build up to a high enough level. This level varies from bird to bird. You can assist the bird by making your aviary unfriendly to the conditions that assist the organisms to thrive. Some suggestions:

- Keep the floor dry. Organisms love moisture as they can dehydrate easily. Check the slope of the floor, which should provide good drainage. Incline the floor slightly so that the water runs off and does not collect in pools. Have a floor that is easy to clean and remove the remnants of food and droppings.
- Do not allow food particles to build up on the floor. These act as food for organisms as well. We know that moist food such as fruit, bread, vegetables and nectar spoils and becomes contaminated if it sits around and is exposed. This contamination is caused by a large build-up of organisms and many of them will be dangerous for the bird. Remove any moist food within 24 hours. Wash and clean all dishes used to provide moist food. Treat the dishes as you would the dishes you eat from. Place them in the dishwasher or wash with detergent each day. Clean up any excess seed and husks regularly, particularly after rain or during humid weather.
- Provide clean, fresh water. Water that is left standing for any long period also develops organisms such as algae and bacteria. It can also become more rapidly contaminated by the presence of food and the bird's droppings. Water should be replaced regularly, preferably each day if it is in an open dish or weekly if in a dropper bottle. The water container should be scrubbed and disinfected at each water change.
- Keep vermin out of the aviary. Vermin carry a number of diseases and can also contaminate food and water by walking through food or depositing urine and faeces into food and water. Rats, mice, cockroaches and wild birds are the main vermin to consider. Other vermin such as owls, foxes, cats and dogs, can cause repeated bouts of stress. Chronic stress can also lower the bird's immune system. Remove or fill any cracks and crevices that provide refuge for vermin. Have a regular vermin control program (baits, traps and insecticides) to remove any vermin before they build up. Seal all food in sturdy storage bins.
- Allow regular exposure to sunlight both for the birds and the aviary. Sunlight is the best disinfectant as it helps dry out organisms. It also has beneficial effects on the bird's health. Avoid overheating and dehydration on hot days by providing shelter and shade.

The Environment

Because you are in charge of the aviary, you have a major input into the bird's environment. You control much of what happens in the environment. Changes to any of the items below can influence what the bird is exposed to and what the organisms are exposed to.

You control:

Food and the food containers
- See the comments on food contamination above.
- The food container can act as a refuge for insects or vermin.
- Food containers can carry poisons (zinc and lead from galvanising).
- Overconsumption of fatty foods (eg sunflower, safflower and nuts) can lead to obesity.
- Poor diets can lead to many nutritional diseases such as vitamin or mineral deficiencies.
- Breeding hens need extra sources of calcium and special soft foods for feeding chicks.
- All-seed diets are deficient in many essential factors.

Water and the water containers
- See the comments on water above.
- Water containers (plastic and galvanised) can leak out poisons.
- Water contaminated with food or droppings can develop high levels of organisms within a few hours on a warm day.
- Position the water container so that moisture is not constantly spilling out to create a moist area close by. This is an excellent means of allowing worm eggs, coccidian oocysts and bacteria to thrive in an area that is regularly walked through by birds. These can then be transmitted to the bird's mouth when it is grooming itself. Overcome this by providing good drainage below and around the water bowl.

Substrate on the floor

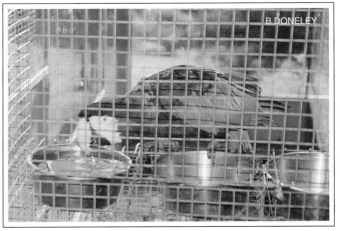

- The substrate can harbour decaying food, insects, worms and other vermin.
- Have a substrate that is easy to clean. Clean it regularly – at least once a week.
- Design the substrate so that it has good drainage. Have it exposed to the sun regularly so that no moist spots develop.
- Avoid the habit of wetting the substrate regularly. In some areas, it is a common

Stainless steel coop cups – ideal feed and water containers – easy to clean, off the ground, and suitable for all sizes.

practice to hose out food and water bowls on the aviary floor every day. This leads to areas that rarely have a chance to dry out – and stops the organisms being dehydrated.
- Design the floor so that any hosing from one floor does not wash into the next aviary and cause cross-contamination.

Materials (wire, walls, shelter, etc) used to construct the aviary
- The choice and design of the aviary can provide refuge for vermin, expose the bird to poisons or expose the bird to extremes of weather and temperature. In Australia the ideal aspect is for your aviary to face north or north-east. Aviaries that face in other directions can allow the birds to be exposed to chilling or overheating. Provide strong barriers (solid walls) particularly to the south and west.
- Remove all tie-wire clippings left over from construction – these are poisonous. Run a magnet over the floor at the end of each day when you are building or renovating.
- Using poor quality galvanised wire will expose the bird to zinc and lead poisoning. Remove all dags from the wire before birds are allowed near it.
- Stainless steel, glass or ceramic containers make the best food and water dishes. Avoid plastic, aluminium, earthenware and galvanised containers.
- Have all wire ties outside the aviary so that birds cannot get caught on them.
- Look at the airflow around and through your aviary. Are the birds exposed to a draught? If you are not sure, take a burning cigarette into each section of the aviary and watch where the smoke trail is drawn. You may need to reposition openings and air-vent holes to avoid problems here. Aim to have a gentle airflow that will keep the birds cool in summer but avoid chilling them in winter.
- Look at the shade that is provided during all seasons. Is it too much or too little?
- Are there enough perches and nestboxes for the bird to feel secure?
- Can a bird escape attention from a bully? Provide visual barriers (eg trees, shrubs, partitions).
- Place nestboxes in a location where they are protected from heat, rain and wind.
- Use materials that minimise injury, escape and theft.
- All solid surfaces should be impervious and easy to clean.
- Use non-toxic (acrylic) paint on all the surfaces that the birds can reach.

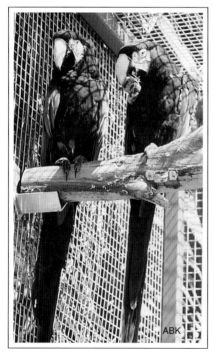

Robust natural perches are absolutely necessary for large parrots like these Green-winged Macaws.

Perches
- Have perches positioned to give the birds the best sense of security. Position them at the highest point in the aviary and under shelter. Avoid placing them close to a metal roof that can become overheated in summer.
- Unsuitable perches can cause feet problems.
- Some materials used may be poisonous. I prefer to use Australian native trees as many of the European trees carry poisons.
- Cracks in perches can provide refuge for some mites.
- Replace the perches regularly, particularly if they are becoming smooth and are not providing adequate grip for the birds.

Protection from weather and many other influences
- Can wild birds (eg Currawongs, butcherbirds, raptors or owls) or other wild animals (eg possums and snakes) access the aviary and harass or pass disease to the residents? Double wiring or solid roofing may be required. Cut back branches that overhang an aviary and provide access for possums, snakes, rats and mice.
- Can dogs or cats approach the aviary so as to

frighten the birds? You may need to provide a solid barrier at the lower aspect of the aviary.

- Is exposure to the wind, rain and sun controlled?

You need to clean the environment regularly. The most important chore is to pick up all the droppings. If you cannot pick them up, then devise a strategy that will cause them to dry out. Normal droppings form a hard crust on the outside that allows the centre to remain moist – this is where the worm eggs and coccidian oocysts survive. Dry concrete floor or sandy substrates which cause the droppings to dry out more quickly are recommended.

The Bird

It is a simple fact that a healthy bird will have a strong immune system that is more capable of fighting disease organisms. What can you do to maintain a bird in as healthy a condition as possible?

- Select good, strong breeding stock. Healthy, strong birds pass this characteristic on to their young.
- Inspect each and every bird daily. Look for departures from the normal. Birds are very good at masking signs of disease. The first signs are often very subtle. The better you know your birds, the more likely you will detect the signs at an early stage.
  - Are the birds eating and drinking?
  - Are the droppings normally formed?
  - Is the bird behaving normally?
  - Is the bird moving and flying normally?
  - Are there any signs of illness?
- Provide the best food available. Malnutrition is a major factor in many birds developing disease. If you are buying seed, fruit and vegetables, buy the best quality you can. Store all foods in ideal conditions away from vermin.
- Many pet birds will be healthier if fed on the new commercial parrot pellet formulations.
- Clean the environment regularly. The area does not need to be sterile but visually clean. As an example, do not feed a bird from a dish that you would not eat from yourself. Use a disinfectant where required. (See the section on *Disinfection* on page 100.)

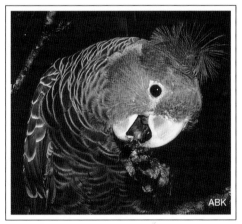

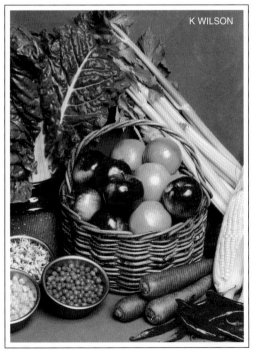

Above: This Gang Gang Cockatoo cock displays all the signs of a normal healthy bird.
Right: Buy the best quality fruit and vegetables.

- Discourage casual visitors from entering your aviary, especially if they have been in contact with another aviary. If you permit them to enter, they must wash their hands and replace their shoes as these are likely to carry organisms from the other aviary.
- Maintain a regular worming program.
- Have a post-mortem performed on any birds that die. This will determine not only why they died, but also answer questions such as:
  - Were there worms present – is your worming program effective?
  - Was the bird overweight – are you feeding correctly?
  - Is the bird in good or poor condition?
  - Was there grit in the gizzard – is the right size and amount being provided and was the bird consuming it?
  - Were the birds sexually active – is there good breeding stimulus and were they a bonded pair?
  - Are there any unexpected problems present?
- Keep stress to a minimum. Stress plays an important role in weakening the bird's immune system. The important principle here is to look at the world through the bird's eyes. Try to imagine what the bird is viewing and how it is responding. You should walk into the aviary and spend some time observing what the bird sees.
- Consider the bird's behavioural requirements:
  - Shy birds need privacy and a secure area to hide if frightened.
  - Flock birds need to have other birds around them – but not in their territory.
  - Most birds do best with one pair to an aviary.
  - Look for signs of bullying or incompatibility in a pair of birds.
  - Spend some time sitting and watching your birds and noting what they are doing and how they are interacting with each other and with their environment. This is best done from a distance. If you are noticed by the birds, they will not behave normally.
- Have a quarantine program.
  - All new birds should be kept separate from your normal aviaries for 4–6 weeks.
  - Refer to the section *How to Set up a Quarantine Program* on page 29.
- If you suspect that a bird is ill, isolate it from other birds and measure its weight. Feel its breast muscles to make sure that the keel bone is not prominent. You can weigh it daily. A bird that is losing weight is in trouble.
- Keep records of all observations of and interactions with the birds. Relying on your memory can trick you. Records should include:
  - Breeding results (mating, egg numbers, hatching numbers, fledging numbers, related birds).
  - Worming treatments (date, medication used, dose, method of administration).
  - Dates of regular pest control measures to eliminate any pests that occur (eg fleas, flies, lice, mites, ticks, mosquitos, rodents).
  - Any diseases and treatments. Record dates to check whether the same problem is recurring each year. Try to devise effective prevention measures.

In summary, disease control comes down to what you do to the birds. You have some influence over the bird, the environment and the organism by how you manage your aviaries. When things go wrong, ask yourself: 'What have I done or not done, that contributed to this?' You need to be your own strongest critic.

Remember, the major way that disease moves around an aviary is via humans – on their hands, feet, clothes and other implements such as buckets and dishes. You need to minimise this.

SO YOU HAVE A SICK BIRD!

At some stage in its life, just as in humans, your bird will develop an illness. This will be an upsetting time as it appears to come on so quickly and you will feel helpless.

People may tell you that there is nothing you can do for a bird when it gets sick. While this may have been true twenty years ago, it is no longer so. There are many new drugs and tests that your veterinarian can use and this seems to expand each day. The secret to curing illness in a bird is to act as soon as signs are visible – because birds hide their signs when they are ill. Most birds that look sick have actually been sick for up to a week but have been hiding their illness.

Later in this book, I have listed some of the more common diseases that you may encounter. My aim is to help you to understand some of the problems that may arise. It is important to realise that many diseases in birds will mimic each other and often the bird will not show any illness until the disease is in an advanced stage. This makes birds one of the most difficult patients to treat and diagnose.

Preservation Reflex

One of the most frustrating problems in avian medicine is the fact that birds do not display illness in the same manner as dogs, cats or the other mammals that we live with. Birds possess the ability to hide most of the symptoms such as lethargy, depression and lack of appetite that we would normally associate with the early stages of a disease process. Many serious illnesses are hidden until the process is quite advanced. This is called the Preservation Reflex. The current theory used to explain this phenomenon is that the birds over the years have developed a reflex action so that they do not show signs of illness. This allows

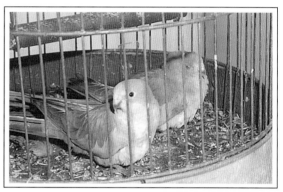

Let's play that new game all aviculturists love – spot the sick bird! Well, they're both quite ill. In fact, we saved the back one and the front one died, despite our best efforts – a great example of the Preservation Reflex.

each bird to preserve itself from attack by predators or to preserve its position in the pecking order.

The significance of this reflex is that simply performing a visual examination of a bird is insufficient to definitely assess its health status. You must pay more attention to small details and make an effort to detect the very subtle, early signs of disease. If a bird displays any signs of illness, this must be acted upon much more quickly than with other pets such as cats and dogs.

By the time birds display signs of illness it is usually a sign that they have reached a stage of decompensation and can no longer mask their illness. They are commonly in an advanced or serious stage of their disease process.

This helps to explain why a bird can be in an advanced state but the owner is convinced that the bird has been ill for only a short period and for the commonly held opinion that birds are 'soft' creatures and die very easily from apparently minor illnesses.

HOW DO I KNOW IF MY BIRD IS SICK?

You need to develop a habit of quickly checking your bird each day. You can monitor the bird quickly and simply by distant examination – ie you don't have to catch the bird. Examine the bird's droppings and look at both the bird and its surrounding environment.

Get to know your bird. Treat any variation from normal habits suspiciously. A common sign of illness is a bird that is sitting in a position in its cage that it normally does not, or allows you to approach closer than normal before showing signs of recognition. Do you know your bird's favourite spots in its cage or how close you approach before it shows signs of recognition? If you don't, you have some work to do.

If you are still concerned that the bird is not normal but cannot put your finger on the cause, trust your intuition. You can do a simple physical examination yourself. Refer to *Signs of Illness* on page 15 for a listing of the common signs of illness and follow the steps in assessing the bird's health. This will act as a guide. If you are concerned, it is wise to take the bird to your veterinarian for a thorough examination and any tests that may be indicated.

Assessing a Bird's Health – the Steps to Recognising Disease

The steps in checking if a bird is healthy are:
1. Examine the droppings.
2. Examine the bird and its environment from a distance.
3. Catch the bird and perform a physical examination.

Examination of Droppings

Do you know what normal droppings from your bird look like? Don't be surprised. Many people don't. It's an area we have been taught to avoid since we were children. Recognition of normal droppings and the range of normal changes is a skill that all bird owners need to develop and check on a daily basis.

The cloaca and vent act as a junction for the contents of the bird's digestive, urinary, and reproductive systems. These are expelled through the 'vent' and are correctly called 'droppings'. A normal dropping should contain excretory products from either the intestine or urinary tract or more commonly both systems.

Normal droppings usually contain:
(a) **From the kidneys** – the urates, a white or creamy paste and the urine, a small amount of watery liquid.
(b) **From the intestines** – the faeces, also called the stool. This is normally a thin coiled tube that may vary in colour.

The colour of the droppings will vary with the pigments in the bird's food or disease. Black, green, brown and brick-red can all be normal colours. Dark coloured faeces may be caused by the presence of blood. Check the bird has not been eating dark pigmented food such as blackberries. Bright green faeces may be a sign of liver disease or blood disorders and are common with malnutrition, toxins, chlamydophila, bacterial septicaemia and some viral diseases. Pale coloured faeces may also be seen with disease of the pancreas or intestine.

A bird's droppings will often give valuable information regarding the state of health. Therefore, it is a good idea to pay close attention to them. Look at the droppings on the floor of the cage – is there an increase or decrease in number compared to what you normally see? Assess both the urinary and faecal components. Expect a temporary increase in urine (the liquid component) due to the excitement of any stress or transport. These wet or liquid droppings are normal after handling or a car trip.

Distant Examination of the Surrounding Environment

Again this is a simple and straightforward technique. Quickly look all around the bird's environment – where it normally lives. While you are doing this, ask yourself the following questions:
• Are there signs of vomiting?
• Are there seed husks on the floor of the cage or in the food container?

- Is the bird eating more of one seed type rather than a mixture?
- Have the other foods (fruit, vegetables etc) been eaten?
- Does the water dish need cleaning?
- Has the bird been chewing the wire or metal components of the cage?
- Are there any other changes to the environment?

Distant Examination of the Bird

Spend a little time observing your bird from a distance, preferably from a location where the bird cannot see you. If you are too close, the bird will respond by hiding any subtle signs of illness. After a minute or so quietly approach the bird and see how it responds to you. Develop a sense for what is normal for each particular bird as there is much individual variation. With practice you can assess your bird very quickly and any departure from normal will be obvious.

A normal bird should display the following:
- Bright and alert behaviour.
- Both eyes wide open and clear with no swelling or discharges.
- Both nostrils open and clear.
- No darkening or stains on feathers near the nostrils.
- It looks at you and responds to your approach.
- Sitting in the normal spots in its cage.
- Standing erect with weight evenly spread on both feet.
- Wings folded against the body in the usual position.
- All feathers are in good condition.
- Moving around actively.
- Singing normally.
- Breathing is barely detectable.
- Not overweight nor very thin.
- No abnormal swellings anywhere on the body.
- No ragged or untidy feathers.

As a general rule of thumb, any caged bird that appears ill to its owner is seriously ill. One day of illness in a small, pet bird is roughly equivalent to one week of illness for a human.

The following list covers some easily recognisable signs that may suggest significant problems for the bird. Any bird with some of the following signs requires close observation and if there is no improvement within 24 hours should be taken to your veterinarian. However, if the bird is huddled and fluffed up, it should be taken to the veterinarian as soon as possible.

SIGNS OF ILLNESS

General Signs
- Weight loss.
- Reduction in appetite or complete cessation of eating.
- Inability to adequately swallow or manipulate food within the mouth.
- Head held under one wing.
- Sitting low down on the perch.
- Vomiting.
- Fluffed feathers – huddled appearance.
- Wet feathers around the head – especially nostrils or eyes.
- Less active than normal – sleepy appearance.
- Droopy wings.
- Decrease in preening activity and maintenance of feathers.
- Broken or untidy feathers.
- A break in the bird's routine indicated by abnormal behaviour.

- Allows you to come closer than normal before responding.
- Cessation of vocalisation.
- Change of voice.
- Visible lumps or masses anywhere on the body.
- Bleeding – always treat this as an emergency.

Eyes
- Discharges from one or both eyes.
- Excessive tears and wetness around the eye.
- Changes in the clarity or colour of eyes.
- Closing of one or both eyes either completely or partially (squinting).
- Swelling around one or both eyes.
- Repeatedly wiping of the head or eyes on the perch.

Nostrils
- Soiling of feathers around the nostrils or of the head feathers.
- Discharges on one or both sides of the nostrils.
- One or both nostrils filled with material.

Respiratory
- Open-mouthed breathing when at rest. Treat this as very serious.
- Tail bobbing when quietly resting, seen as a rhythmic back and forth motion of the tail.
- Sneezing, wheezing or gasping.

Musculoskeletal/Neurological
- Balancing problems, eg falling off the perch or flying erratically.
- Inability to perch. This bird will remain on the bottom of the cage.
- Limping or lack of full weight-bearing on one limb.
- Swollen foot/feet and/or joint/joints.

Droppings
- Change in quantity of droppings.
- Increased water component in droppings.
- Sloppy components and not properly formed.
- Whole seeds are passed in droppings.
- Droppings are stuck to the vent or staining of the feathers near the vent or tail.

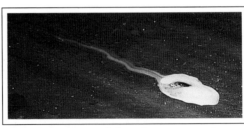

The sloppiness of this dropping is due to excess urates not the faeces, so this is called polyuria, not diarrhoea, and is a sign of kidney disease.

Asleep or a Sick Bird?
A common question people ask about observing birds is: 'How do you tell the difference between a bird that is asleep and one that is sick?' On first look these conditions can be very similar – the bird will be huddled, with its head under one wing and the feathers fluffed. Use the following signs to help tell them apart:

A Bird that is Asleep
- During the day it is more common for birds to be asleep in mid-morning and early mid-afternoon.
- Birds often sleep with only one foot on the perch, the other raised.
- The bird will be easily aroused with only a slight sound.
- Once awake, the bird will:
  - Tighten its feathers, stretch its wings and be quite alert.

- Open its eyes widely.
- Become active and behave normally.
- Wings will be held in the normal position, with the wing tips touching as they normally would.

A 'Sick' Bird

- The bird will be in a sleeping position at most times of the day, particularly when other birds are active.
- The bird will have both feet on the perch, often with a crouched posture.
- The bird is not as easily roused, is less alert and allows you to come closer than normal before trying to escape.
- Once awake, the bird:
  - May have slightly closed eyes, as if squinting.
  - Sits quietly for a short time, then adopts a sleeping position once again.
- Often the bird will be found in an unusual location in the aviary or cage, eg sitting on the floor.
- The wings may be drooping, with the wing tips in an abnormal position.
- Look for other signs of illness:
  - Abnormal behaviour.
  - Sloppy droppings.
  - Vomiting or groups of seed stuck together on the floor or walls.
  - A decreased number of droppings.
  - Not eating its food or eating too much.
  - Not drinking water.
  - Drinking too much water.
  - Sneezing or strange sounds when breathing.
  - Heavy breathing (tail bobbing).
  - Brown stained feathers above the nostrils.
  - Discharge from eyes or nostrils.
  - Abnormal moulting.
  - Excessive picking at feathers.

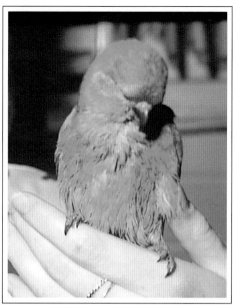

Typical signs of a sick bird in a Musk Lorikeet.

HOW TO DO A PHYSICAL EXAMINATION

This is a summary of the simple features you need to check. It will not replace a thorough examination by your veterinarian. I include it so that you can perform some simple aspects yourself and can see the complexity of the beginning of a thorough physical examination that your veterinarian will use to help diagnose the problems that may be found in a bird.

- I prefer to start at the head and move down the body. Place particular emphasis on any suggestive signs detected during the distant examination.
- Examine the head, eyes, ears, nostrils and cere. Pay particular attention to the feathers immediately adjacent to the nostrils as even a mild discharge will make dust adhere to them and give them a stained appearance. This is the equivalent of a runny nose. The head should be symmetrical. Examine the head on top, from the front and

back and each side, looking for any asymmetry. Examine the beak for damage or malformation. Bruising of the beak may be associated with liver disease or trauma.

- Open the mouth and examine the tongue, choana (the slit in the roof of the mouth) and throat. Note any sour or abnormal odours. Is there excessive mucous or cheesy plaque present? Examine the fringe lining the choana. In chronic respiratory disease or Vitamin A deficiency, the fringe will be damaged or missing.
- Carefully run your fingers over the entire bird, beginning at the crop and working down the keel to the abdomen.
- The crop may contain food but rarely fluid. In aviary birds the crop will be empty in the middle of the day as they eat early in the day and late in the evening similar to birds in the wild. Pet birds will often eat all day. In a young bird delayed crop emptying is often the first sign of disease.
- The oesophagus passes down the right side of the neck and is usually thin walled unless the parents are feeding young.
- The breast muscles should be convex and the keel bone should not be prominent. (This does not apply to very young birds who are not yet flying or flightless birds such as quail, Ostrich or Emu.)
- The abdomen should be concave (slightly sunken) not convex. The lower abdominal contents are often easily examined. The gizzard is found in the lower left quadrant. Usually if the liver edge (most easily found on the right) can be felt, it is enlarged. If the abdomen is enlarged, examination must be extremely gentle. The bird should not demonstrate pain with a normal, gentle abdominal examination.
- Examine the vent for swellings, encrustations or soiling, indicative of loose droppings. If the tail is gently flexed towards the back, the vent will open and allow inspection of the cloaca.
- Examine the feathers and skin. Look for any missing or chewed feathers. Are any feathers damaged or malformed – particularly the primary flight and tail feathers? In pigeons and parrots, part the feathers over the hip and closely examine the powder down feathers (these are not present in most other commonly kept birds). Are the powder down feathers fluffy and is it difficult to see the skin beneath or are they thin and deformed? Does the bird have a powder covering on all the feathers and beak? Lack of powder and a shiny beak may be an early sign of Psittacine Beak and Feather Disease (PBFD).
- Pull out each wing individually. Feel the bones from the shoulder to the wing tip. Examine each joint for full range of motion or any swelling. Hold each wing up to a bright light to transilluminate the feathers. Spray methylated spirits on the skin if closer inspection is required. This may reveal bruising of a swollen area.
- Examine each leg individually. Run your fingers from the hip to the end of each claw, paying particular attention to the joints.
- Assess the gripping ability of each toe. A weak grip may indicate abdominal tumours, fractures or disease of the nervous system.
- Lameness of one leg is more common than both legs. Is the bird placing more weight on one leg and favouring the other?
- Assess the length of the claws. Overgrown claws may be associated with liver disease, nutritional problems or poor perches.
- Inspect the bottom of each foot. The surface should be rough, not smooth. A smooth surface at the base of the foot may be the first sign of incorrect perching material or the beginning of 'bumble foot'.
- Once the examination is finished immediately place the bird back into its cage and assess its tolerance of the procedure. Most birds will look normal and many will preen themselves to reposition any feathers ruffled by your hand. If the bird looks obviously stressed or is breathing heavily, assume it is ill.

HOW TO MAKE YOUR VISIT TO THE VETERINARIAN MORE SUCCESSFUL

To enable the veterinarian to get the most out of his/her examination and to help the bird to travel well, follow these directions:

- Any ill bird should be taken to your veterinarian as soon as possible. The sooner a bird is examined and a diagnosis achieved, the more likely it will respond well to treatment.
- Remove any swings, toys etc in a cage that may move around and injure the bird during transportation.
- If it is cold or windy, cover the cage to protect the bird.
- Bring the bird in the cage it normally lives in or in the cage it is presently living in if that is different.
- Do not clean the cage prior to the veterinarian visit. Place newspaper or Glad Wrap™ on the floor of the cage to allow collection of good samples of droppings for tests. Leave all food dishes as they are. Leave any vomitus, diarrhoea etc.
- Remove the water dish and empty it before transportation so that it does not spill and change the character of any droppings.
- Take any medications or treatments that have been used. Remember to tell your veterinarian ALL the medications you have used or it will lead to confusion in the diagnosis and interpretation of laboratory tests. Any antibiotics given within 48 hours may interfere with laboratory results. If the veterinarian is aware that medication has been used, it allows them to consider test results more accurately.
- Make sure that the bird is accompanied by someone who knows the current history. If you are unable to attend have a telephone contact available, or provide a detailed written history.

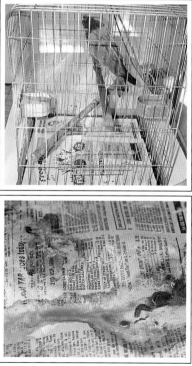

- A live bird is more useful for diagnosing disease. If the bird is likely to die make every effort to take it to your veterinarian while it is still alive so that samples of blood and body fluids are fresh. Some diseases that can be diagnosed in a live bird are much harder to diagnose in a dead one.
- If the bird dies it is best if it is taken to your veterinarian within six hours. If this is not possible, you can help to preserve the bird in good condition by wetting it thoroughly as soon after death as possible. A few drops of liquid detergent added to the water helps to soak the feathers more effectively. Wrap the wet bird in 2–3 layers of Glad Wrap™ and place it in the refrigerator – NOT THE FREEZER. This can help preserve the bird for up to a week, although as time passes the tissues will deteriorate. The sooner this is done after death, the longer the bird will last before it begins to deteriorate.
- Transport the dead bird to your veterinarian in a container that will keep it cool.

FIRST AID

Any bird showing signs of illness must be treated as an emergency. If the bird has been ill, but not showing signs because of its preservation reflex, by the time it is showing signs of being ill it will be dehydrated and often will have a low temperature

Top: Bird in cage – note the newspaper on the base.
Bottom: Abnormal droppings on paper.

(hypothermia). A bird in this condition is heading towards shock and kidney failure. All first aid must be guided by the principle: 'Do No Harm'.

It is a common approach in aviculture to give antibiotics to any sick bird or to give antibiotics regularly to prevent illness. Both these techniques can cause more problems than they solve. Antibiotics are only a useful treatment for diseases caused by bacteria. There is no antibiotic that will treat all bacteria. Before you give antibiotics to your bird you need to be certain that the disease is one that is caused by bacteria and that the antibiotic you are using is the correct one for this situation and that you are using the correct dosage.

A better approach to a sick bird is to help it fight the problems you know are developing, such as shock and/or kidney failure. The most reliable means of doing this is to give fluid therapy and support the bird's needs.

Fluid Therapy – Electrolytes

These are a simple but very effective aid for all sick birds. If I have to make a choice between giving a sick bird an antibiotic and giving it some electrolytes, I would choose the electrolytes as my first attack on disease.

Because birds are very poor at showing that they are ill, until they are in an advanced stage, they all are beginning to suffer from dehydration when it is finally apparent that they do have a problem. Unless this dehydration is treated, they will ultimately die. Electrolyte mixes given via a crop needle or directly to the beak are an excellent way of helping reverse the effects of dehydration and give the bird strength to fight off the effects of disease.

These electrolyte solutions are available from nearly every veterinarian in Australia. They are designed for use in other domestic animals but are equally useful for birds. Common brands are Lectade™,

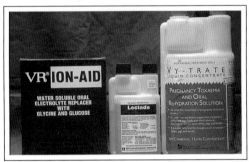

Examples of some of the common electrolytes that are extremely useful in any ill bird.

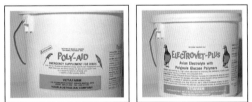

Vytrate™, Ion-Aid™, Electrovet™, Polyaid™. In an emergency, you can use sports drinks such as Gatorade™ and Sports Plus™, or electrolytes from the chemist such as Gastrolyte™ or Lucozade™. These also have glucose in them which helps give the bird a burst of energy as well as fighting the dehydration. Mix according to the directions on the packet and administer in the drinking water as well as giving fluids equivalent to 10% of the bird's body weight directly into the crop (or very carefully into the beak).

Examples:
- A Budgerigar weighing 50 grams would be given 5ml spread throughout the day – 0.5ml at a time.
- A Galah weighing 300 grams would be given 30ml spread throughout the day – 4 to 5ml at a time.

Ideal Environment for A Sick Bird
- Isolation stops the bird from feeling threatened and helps reduce the chance of disease transmission to other birds.
- Warmth. A warm place in the sun is not enough. Use a hospital cage or similar to give the bird a stable temperature of 28–30°C. But this must be a moist, humid warmth or you will merely help dehydrate the bird more quickly. Aim for a humidity of

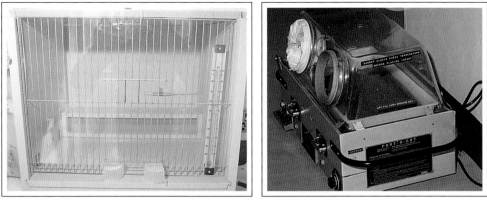

A hospital cage and humidicrib used for housing sick birds.

approximately 70%. The best way to achieve this is to provide a shallow dish of water, covered to prevent accidental drowning and drinking, or wet cottonwool in a dish in the enclosure with a reliable thermostat attached to the heat source (that does not allow temperature fluctuations of more than 1°C). It is best to have a reliable thermometer and hygrometer inside the enclosure as close as possible to where the bird will be sitting so it is measuring the environment where the bird actually is. It is not uncommon to see these instruments positioned at the top of the cage where they are actually measuring different temperatures and humidity to that which is found where the bird is sitting. Observe the bird for signs to adjust the temperature control. If the bird is too hot, it will pant and stretch its neck while holding its wings away from its body. If it is too cold, it will remain huddled and hunched with its feathers fluffed. Be prepared to adjust the control until the bird looks more normal.

- Easy access to food and water. Most sick birds will sit on the bottom of the cage and not move. Place the food and water dishes close to the bird so it is encouraged to use them. Use electrolytes in the water and provide food that is easily digested such as fruit and vegetables. Remember that the environment is quite warm so you will need to replace the water and food as it becomes warm as it may be less palatable. Many parrots will eat peanut butter on toast when they reject all other foods. This gives them a burst of energy and helps maintain their metabolism. If birds stop eating, their body temperature begins to drop. To avoid this you may need to force feed them. Use of a crop needle can be a life saver.

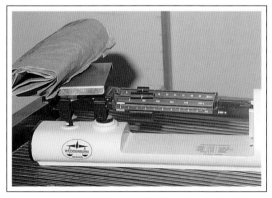

A bird wrapped in a butcher's bag and placed on balance beam scales. Electronic scales are more modern but these are useful and still quite accurate.

Weighing Your Bird

Using a set of scales to weigh your sick bird each day, is an excellent means of monitoring the progress. If the bird is gaining weight, you are winning and the treatment should be maintained. If it is losing weight, then you are losing and you need to change your approach. If the weight is stable, then you need to keep on with the treatment, but reassess your diagnosis if the weight does not improve within 48 hours.

To make the weighing exercise more accurate, weigh the bird at the same time each day. The best time is early in the day, before any medication is given.

PURCHASING YOUR FIRST BIRD

When you first decide to purchase a bird, you need to give some thought as to the best way to prevent any diseases or problems arising in this new bird. Only purchase birds that are fit, healthy and active. While this will not totally rule out disease problems, it makes it more likely you will not introduce disease into your aviary.

If the bird is valuable, it should be taken to your veterinarian for a thorough examination and testing. Your veterinarian will perform an examination and tests designed to detect any diseases that may cause health or breeding problems. The tests that are commonly performed are designed to detect chlamydophilosis, intestinal parasites and bacterial infections. With expensive birds, blood tests and X-rays may be used as well.

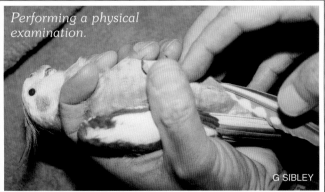

Performing a physical examination.

G SIBLEY

If you are unable to take your bird to your veterinarian, follow these steps:

1. Perform a distant examination of the bird. Look for the signs of disease as listed previously.
2. Perform a distant examination of the environment.
3. Pay particular attention to the bird's droppings.
4. Catch the bird and perform a physical examination.

If any abnormal signs are present, take the bird to your veterinarian to give you an opinion before you finalise the purchase of the bird. This should be discussed with the person who is selling the bird to you.

ANNUAL HEALTH EXAMINATION FOR PET BIRDS

There is a trend for avian veterinarians to recommend that a pet bird have an annual health examination. This has been a regular event in North America and is beginning to become more popular in Australia.

Why should you bother? The answer is simple. Birds mask the signs of illness so a bird that looks normal may actually have low grade disease problems present. These will only be detected if you check for them. In addition, many of the major causes of death in pet birds are a result of a preventable disease or one that could have been easily treated if detected sooner. These include malnutrition, end stage organ failure (especially pancreas, liver, kidney and heart) and behavioural problems such as screaming and biting. Acute illnesses are much less common but should also be included in the examination, particularly with a new pet.

There is a definite trend in human medicine to use regular tests to detect problems at an early stage. This is well established for diseases such as breast cancer, cervical cancer (PAP smears) and prostate cancer. It is recommended that you use the same principle to test your pet bird for some of the more common problems they can develop.

There is also a trend to include an observation and discussion of the bird's behaviour and to use this to provide advice on shaping the bird's behaviour so that it can adapt to the household better and become a happier pet. Behavioural problems are a major cause of stress for both the bird and its owner and are a common cause of the bird being relocated to a new home. Some time spent addressing these issues can relieve a lot of this stress.

Preventative medicine is applicable to all animals and begins when you first acquire your new pet. The new pet should have a thorough examination to detect any problems that may be present. It is recommended that you repeat the health examination each year.

The first part of the examination involves a discussion of what is happening with the bird. Topics will include diet, levels of activity and behavioural issues such as how the bird interacts with people and any problems that may be developing.

A thorough physical examination is then conducted. The bird is also weighed. As birds are experts at masking the signs of illness, this will cover many of the different organ systems.

Finally, some samples may be taken for examination in the laboratory. These may include samples of the bird's droppings, as well as swabs from the bird's mouth and vent. A full blood count and biochemical profile may also be performed. Crop washes are necessary in some species. In some cases samples may be examined using DNA analysis to detect *Chlamydophila psittaci* and some of the serious viral diseases. These tests may be expensive and are not suitable or necessary for everyone. Your avian veterinarian will discuss your needs with you to gauge what suits your bird and your situation.

An annual health examination is an excellent means of identifying problems at an early stage and treating them before they develop into a major issue.

HINTS ON KEEPING BIRDS IN CAPTIVITY

Hygiene Procedures

Hygiene is simply using good housekeeping techniques to prevent disease building up in your aviary. Is a dirty aviary acceptable? At first consideration this seems to be a fairly straightforward question but it really is quite complex. Dirt in itself is quite inoffensive. Every day people and animals are exposed to dirt. So where is the problem? Well, the real problem is contamination. Disease results when the number of disease organisms are able to overwhelm the birds' defences and so they become sick. Contamination is an unseen hazard. Disease organisms can be excreted in most body fluids – saliva, sneeze droplets, vomit, eye secretions rubbed onto perches and most importantly in the droppings. So all your efforts should be aimed to remove the build-up of these.

A healthy bird is usually able to cope with a significant number of disease organisms before it succumbs. On the other hand a stressed or weak bird will succumb to a much lower number of organisms, because its immune system is weakened. So disease prevention is really a combination of keeping the number of disease organisms down to a level that the bird can live with and to keep the bird strong and protected so its immune system is 100% and can fight disease.

How do you control contamination? The best guide is to keep the aviary as clean as

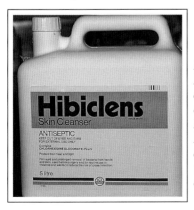

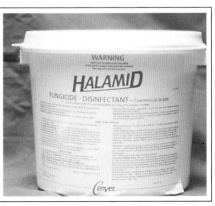

Left: Hibiclens™, a very useful disinfectant. Right: Halamid™, another useful disinfectant.

you would your own house. Clean up any soft food (fruit, vegetables, greens, cake etc) daily. Keep all dishes that contain food and water cleaned regularly. Treat any dishes that contain moist foods as you would a dish you were using at the dinner table – clean them daily in a dishwasher or detergent. Clean up the droppings and spilled seed once a week.

If you cannot remove the droppings, use a rake or broom to break up the pellets of droppings. This allows the centre of the pellet to dry out. The major cause of worm eggs and bacteria surviving is moisture. For the same reason you should design the floor of the aviary to minimise the build-up of moisture. A major problem site is around the water dish. The build-up of droppings and moisture is a lethal combination. Use a good flow-over drain or rubble to allow all moisture to drain away quickly. Have the floor sloping to decrease flat spots where moisture can collect.

Disinfectants can be useful, but their use must be strictly according to the manufacturer's instructions. Don't rely on them to work miracles. As a rule of thumb, disinfection is 90% perspiration and elbow grease and 10% chemical. For all disinfectants, you need to get in and clean the area well so that it is visibly clean, then apply the disinfectant that has been accurately made up and leave it on for the recommended amount of time. If you leave some droppings or seed husks or food on the area it will inactivate the disinfectant and you will achieve almost nothing.

The safest disinfectants to use around birds are bleach (chlorine), chloramine, tertiary amines, chlorhexidine and quaternary ammonium compounds. (For more information refer to *Disinfection* on page 100.)

Other disinfectants such as phenolics, formaldehydes and glutaraldehyde are useful but can be dangerous to people or birds if they come into contact with them. These can be used but you need to take a lot of care with them and rinse extremely well after use. Look on the label of your favourite disinfectant and find the active ingredient to see which it contains.

Stress Control

Stress is a normal and natural phenomenon. It only becomes a problem when the bird cannot cope or escape from the cause. You need to know your birds' needs well enough to suspect that stress may be a problem.

Common causes of stress are:
• Excessive noise that is not normally present.
• Presence of predators such as cats, dogs, foxes etc.
• Disturbance at night from rats, mice, owls etc.
• Poor protection from extremes of weather.
• Lack of food or water.
• Dietary deficiencies.
• Bullying from other birds.
• Lack of exercise.
• Poor shelter.

The basic step to avoiding stress is to provide a secure aviary where:
• The birds know they can escape from predators.
• People don't enter other than during your normal routines for feeding and cleaning.
• There is provision of an adequate and palatable, balanced diet.
• There is provision of plenty of perches and nesting sites.
• There are visual barriers so birds can escape from their mate or others if there is fighting.
• There is good protection from winds and rain and chilling.
• Rodent and other vermin/pest control is adequate.
• Contamination is reduced to a viable level.
• Good levels of exercise are available and encouraged.

Disease Prevention

This begins with a quarantine period for each and every bird that comes onto your premises. I know that this bird is the one you have saved for and wanted and now that it is finally here you are desperate to get it into the aviary and begin breeding. This is a recipe for disaster. Develop a little patience and keep the bird separate from all your other birds. Allow it time to settle into the new premises, to become accustomed to your face and your diet and daily routine. During this time worm it twice, or preferably have the droppings tested as well. Also, check the bird for lice, mites or other obvious signs of disease.

I don't routinely recommend the use of antibiotics during the quarantine period, except in the case of birds such as young Neophema Grass Parrots or Budgerigars, which are so prone to developing Psittacosis that a course of doxycycline (eg Psittavet™) should be given for 42 days. Remember that Psittacosis is an extremely contagious disease and that even if it doesn't affect your birds, it can affect you and the members of your family.

An important principle to understand is that the use of drugs to control disease is similar to using Band-aids™ – patching up the problem after it has arisen. If possible it is better to anticipate disease and to head it off. An important part of any disease prevention program is the decision to learn from each disease outbreak and to try to change your management techniques (ie anything that you do with your birds) to try to prevent the problem arising again. You need to put some time aside and ask yourself the question: 'What can I change about the way that I look after my birds to stop this happening again?' Such questions should include:

- Do you need to clean the floor more often?
- Do you need to change the way you store your feed?
- Do you need to worm your birds more regularly or at more appropriate times of the year?
- Do you need to get rid of the mealworm colony in the floor of your aviary because they are a reservoir for tapeworms?
- Do you need to change the diet?
- Do you need to change your nestboxes more frequently?

These and many other questions will vary from aviculturist to aviculturist. You need to be very hard on yourself and be very critical of your methods, but the experience is well worth the effort. Seek the help of experienced aviculturists and avian veterinarians to solve your problems.

Some important disease prevention hints are:

- To control roundworm and *Capillaria*, keep the birds away from their droppings as much as possible. If there is a wet spot on the floor of your aviary use a wire

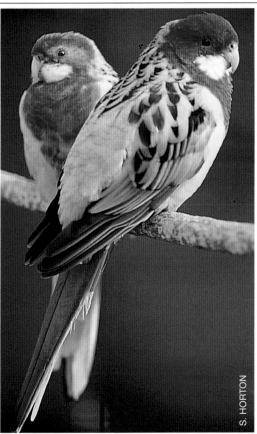

Golden-mantled Eastern Rosellas showing signs of illness.

covering or change the floor to remove it. Remember, moist areas on the floor help more worm eggs to survive.

- To control gizzardworm and tapeworm, use Coopex™ around your aviary to control the insects that can carry the intermediate stage of these worms.
- Prevent wild birds having access to your aviaries.
- Don't use a compost on the floor of your aviary as a source of insect food as it provides a home for other insects that can carry diseases, such as tapeworm.
- Store your seed in sealed drums to protect the seed from pests such as mice, rats, sparrows and insects.
- Quarantine ALL newly purchased birds.
- Keep records of diseases you have had in the past and any treatment that was successful.

Converting your Pet Bird to a Commercial Pelleted Diet

Why should you bother with changing your pet parrot's diet? It is a regular observation by avian veterinarians that many parrots develop health problems because they are eating too high a level of fat in their diet combined with an unbalanced intake of protein, vitamins and minerals. The traditional seed-based diets that are offered appear to suit aviary birds much more than the pet that lives in the house with people.

Parrots are intelligent animals and they resent any changes to their lifestyle – especially when you attempt to change their diet. In this regard, they are rather like people and they love their food. They will not eat any new foods because they simply do not recognise them as food and they are waiting for you to provide them with their regular diet.

Birds that have converted to a pelleted diet should always be given variety by supplementing the pellets with small amounts of other foods such as fruit, vegetables, cooked meat, bread and nuts. You can offer your bird a small amount of what you are eating. Some birds such as Cockatiels do well if offered 2–3 sunflower seeds each day. This small number of sunflower seeds is good for the bird, but any more can be unhealthy. Any of these treats should be offered to the bird in a clean food bowl, separate to the bowl containing the pellets. The bowl containing the treats should be removed after 4–6 hours, before they spoil.

Always have fresh water provided daily. Birds eating pellets often consume more water than those on seed diets, so you need a bowl that contains a sufficient volume of water.

Getting started
- A diet change should only be attempted with a healthy bird. If you are unsure, have your avian veterinarian check your bird's health before beginning this process.
- Weigh the bird and record it in a book. This is the weight that you want the bird to maintain as you change the diet. Use this weight as a guide to check how successful you are.
- Reweigh the bird at the same time each morning for two weeks. Record the weight in your book to monitor your progress. If the bird is losing weight,

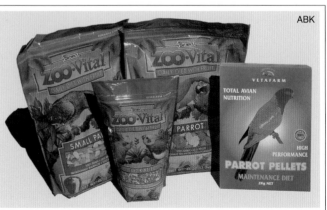

Some of the pelleted food available to aviculturists.

you need to try some of the tips below. If your bird loses a lot of weight take it to your avian veterinarian for a health check.

- Place the pellets in the usual feeding dish. This is where the bird expects to find food.
- To begin, mix the pellets 50:50 with the regular food. As the bird begins to eat the mix, gradually reduce the amount of the regular food over the next few weeks. Take it slowly. There is no rush, particularly if the bird is maintaining its normal weight.
- Expect the bird to throw tantrums and scream at you – they really are creatures of habit and are resistant to any change – this is normal. Talk to your bird in a calm voice – do not scream back, no matter how frustrated you feel.

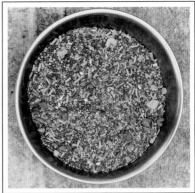

An ideal way to introduce birds to pellets is to mix pelleted food with their regular seed.

Some successful tips when the bird will not eat the pellets
- Place the pellets in a bowl near the highest perch, as most birds prefer to eat from the highest bowl first.
- Let the bird see you pretending to eat the food or another bird eating the food – they love to mimic others.
- Crush the pellets and sprinkle some over the bird's favourite food (eg its favourite fresh fruit) so that the bird will take in a mouthful of pellets when it eats the food. Over-ripe or very soft fruit works best as it is stickier and the pellets adhere more easily. Do not leave this type of food in the cage more than 4–6 hours as it spoils very easily.
- Give the bird the normal food for only 30 minutes morning and night. This allows their appetite to develop. Place the pellets in the normal bowl for the rest of the time so that the bird can eat them as a snack.
- Mix the regular seed and the pellets 50:50 in a bowl. Add small amounts of hot water until you have a sticky consistency. Mix it together in your hands and roll it into small rissoles about 1–2cm in diameter. Place these fresh rissoles in the bird's normal food bowl. Make these rissoles every day but gradually reduce the amount of seed.
  To make the rissoles more attractive, you can roll them in a bowl of seed to form a coating on the outside.
- Mix the pellets 50:50 with soaked seed – this is especially useful when the hen is rearing her young as she is more likely to take in strange food that is moist for the chicks.
- Add the pellets to a scoop of peanut butter and offer it from your hand.

If nothing is working
- Remove all perches from the cage so that the bird has to sit on the edge of the food dish.
- Board your bird with an avian veterinarian. This is often more successful as the bird is easier to switch its diet when it is away from the comfort of its normal surroundings. Veterinarians are experienced in weighing the bird and monitoring its health.

Sprouted Seeds

Sprouted seeds are a treat for many birds and are commonly used when the parents are feeding chicks. When the seeds are sprouted, they become a source of protein and energy that is more easily digested than the dry seed.

There have been disease problems and deaths associated with sprouted seeds, as dangerous bacteria have been found in some batches. Some simple changes to the way

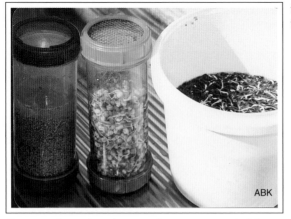

Sprouted seed and mung beans, essential in a balanced nutritional diet.

the seeds are sprouted can avoid the build-up of these bacteria.

- Use only glass or stainless steel bowls for soaking and sprouting, as they are more effectively disinfected prior to use. Plastic is porous and harbours bacteria in any cracks. Plastic is safe until it becomes contaminated and then it can be a disaster. You can certainly use plastic, but it will eventually let you down.
- Use only seed that is top quality and clean. Try this simple test. Count out 100 seeds. Soak and sprout them. If over 80% of them do not sprout, they are a poor batch.
- Do not use dusty or dirty seed as it is more likely to contain bacteria.
- Some seed can be infected with a fungus. This is more likely with seed that has been grown in irrigated pastures. It is more common in sunflower, safflower, millet, corn, peanuts and some grains. Spreading the seed out on a cloth or clean tarpaulin and exposing it to the sun for several hours can reduce the fungus prior to sprouting.
- There are two basic seed groups:
  1. *Oil seeds*. These are high in energy and protein and easy to sprout. The birds find them palatable, so they are readily accepted as a food source. They include sunflower, safflower, rape, lettuce, niger, linseed, nuts (eg peanuts, almonds) and all the pulses and legumes (eg alfalfa, tic beans, mung beans, lentils, chick peas, broad beans, dun peas, maple peas, black-eyed peas, split peas, kidney beans, soybeans, lupins). They are suitable for feeding to parents prior to hatching and to the young when they have fledged. Many legumes (eg soybeans, lupins) are not fed raw as they contain natural poisons. However, these can be inactivated by cooking them (boiling in fresh water until they are soft).

     Note: Almonds will not sprout, but will swell and become softer. Some seeds, such as niger, will not sprout without special laboratory conditions.
  2. *Starch seeds*. These are high in energy but lower in protein. They include cereals (eg maize, barley, wheat, oats and milo), pannicum, canary seed and the millets (eg Red, French White, Japanese). These are offered to parents feeding their young.
- Different seeds take different times to germinate, eg Japanese millet, rape and pannicum sprout quickly, but canary is much slower.
- If you follow the recommended process you will minimise the problems with feeding soaked seed:
  1. Do not use water from the tap or hose, as it may contain bacteria. Use distilled water that has been boiled and allowed to cool, or use water that contains a weak solution of chlorhexidine (eg 1:1000 Aviclens™).
  2. Sterilise the soaking container with a reliable disinfectant. Use a glass or stainless steel container.
  3. Before soaking, clean the seed by rinsing it in disinfectant, eg 0.5ml bleach (sodium hypochlorite) per litre of water.
  4. Soak the seed for 12 hours by immersing in enough water to fully cover it.
  5. After 12 hours, drain the water from the seed and rinse it thoroughly at least 4 or 5 times or until the water is clean. The seed should have a clean, sweet odour. If it has an offensive odour, discard it and start again.

6. Leave the seed in the container after all the water has been drained. Enough water should remain to keep it moist.
7. Repeat the draining and cleaning twice a day.
8. When a green shoot protrudes from the seed it is ready to feed to the birds. This will occur on the third day in most cases.
9. Before feeding the seed to the birds, rinse it thoroughly and then soak it for 10 minutes in a weak solution of chlorhexidine (eg 1:1000 Aviclens™).
10. Give the bird the sprouted seed on a clean dish. Any sprouted seed not eaten by the birds within 12 hours should be thrown away.

HOW TO SET UP
A QUARANTINE PROGRAM

The aim of quarantine is to prevent any disease from entering your premises and infecting your other birds. As well, it is used to monitor the bird during its settling in time as this is the time when any disease it may be carrying is most likely to break out. The recommended quarantine time is a minimum of four weeks, although up to six weeks would be preferable. Even if you have a veterinary examination prior to purchase and the bird is deemed healthy, a quarantine period should still be carried out.

All birds are surrounded by organisms that can possibly cause infections. Usually their immune system can cope with this well and will stop any disease from taking hold. Prior to reaching its new home the bird will have been stressed. Simply moving a bird to new premises can be stressful for them. This means that any disease it has been carrying that was controlled by its immune system can break out. Many birds appear healthy but are actually 'carriers' of disease. Also, any disease the bird has been exposed to on the way or in the new premises can be a serious threat.

The best advice is to begin with as healthy a bird as possible. Follow the guidelines for examining a bird and assessing its health as set out earlier. All new birds should be examined thoroughly.

During the quarantine period you need to take some preventative steps to reduce stress. The area you use to quarantine new birds should be as far away as possible from your aviaries and other birds. It should have separate food and water dishes that are never taken over to the normal aviary areas. It should be an area that is not brightly lit and in as quiet a location as possible. Introduce the new bird to the quarantine cage as early in the day as possible. This gives it a chance to settle down and locate the food and water dishes and a safe, secure perch for the night.

If there is more than one bird, make sure that there are enough dishes and perches to avoid fighting. Have enough perches at the highest point in the cage, for all birds to comfortably roost for the night. Birds instinctively roost in the highest point possible and will fight over a perch if there are not enough available. Spend some time observing the birds to detect any signs of aggression or bullying. Any fighting will add to the stress and should be avoided. Some birds are incompatible and cannot be kept together.

During the quarantine time:
• The birds should be wormed at least twice. If possible, have their droppings tested by your veterinarian.
• Australian parrots that may have been exposed to Psittacosis should be given a six-week course of Doxycycline (Psittavet™). With *Polytelis* or *Neophema* species which are extremely sensitive to Psittacosis, this should be done as a routine procedure.

Preventative Treatments

In the following birds there are diseases which may need preventative treatment. Discuss this with your veterinarian. The drugs listed are the most effective treatments currently. This will change with time and your location.

Coccidiosis: In Budgerigars, finches, pigeons, quail, pheasants use Baycox™, Coccivet™ or Amprolmix Plus™.

Trichomoniasis: In Budgerigars and some cockatoos, canaries and pigeons use Emtryl™, Flagyl™, Metrin™, Torgyl™, Spartrix™ or Ronivet S™.

Scaly-face Mite: In Budgerigars, Neophemas, canaries and Kakarikis use Ivomec™ or Cydectin™.

MEDICATING BIRDS

How to Use a Gavage (Crop) Needle

This technique can mean the difference between a sick bird surviving or dying. It is a technique that everyone who keeps birds needs to be able to perform. While most veterinarians will use this technique to collect samples from the crop to diagnose disease, it is also useful for handrearing, medicating birds that are ill, or for giving medications such as worming mixtures, to prevent disease.

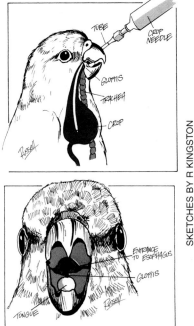

SKETCHES BY R KINGSTON

For birds with a strong bite, particularly parrots, use a stainless steel gavage (crop) needle. The most useful size for parrots is 14–18 gauge and 100–150mm long. For other birds, a soft plastic or rubber tube may be used. These are attached to a syringe containing the appropriate amount of medication.

For a right-handed person the technique is as follows. (If you are left-handed, reverse the directions as appropriate).

1. Hold the bird in your left hand.
2. Adjust the tension you use to hold the bird until it is comfortable and ceases struggling. If the bird is held too loosely or too tightly it will struggle.
3. Use the tips of your fingers to stretch the neck so that the beak is uppermost.
4. Hold the syringe so that you can roll it between two fingers, your index finger and thumb, similar to holding a pen. ONLY USE TWO FINGERS WHEN ROLLING IT.
5. Never force the gavage needle. Use twisting and rolling movements between your two fingers to allow it to slide down.

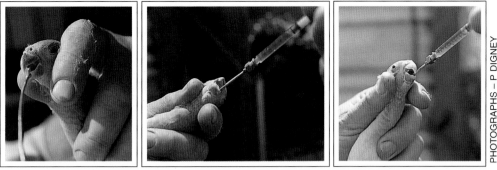

PHOTOGRAPHS – P DIGNEY

Left: Enter from the bird's left side.
Centre: Once behind the tongue, lift the needle up and ease down the neck.
Right: By feeling the tip against your thumb you can gauge the depth. Slowly administer the solution.

6. Place the tip of the needle on the left side of the bird's beak.
7. Gently twist and roll the ball so that it passes over the tongue. Aim towards your thumb and the back of the bird's throat.
8. Gently slide the tip of the gavage needle towards the right side of the bird's mouth. Minimal pressure is required.
9. Pass the needle down the side of the mouth. The area you want to avoid pushing the needle into is called the glottis – the entrance to the windpipe. It is located in the centre of the mouth at the base of the tongue. If the needle is passed down the side of the mouth, it should avoid the glottis and the windpipe.
10. It is usually easy to tell if you enter the windpipe. The bird will stop screaming at you and you will feel a small bumping sensation that is caused by the needle passing over the rings of cartilage that line the windpipe.
11. As the needle leaves the mouth, raise the angle of the syringe. Now, aim straight down the side of the bird's neck, alongside or parallel to your thumb. Gently direct the needle down the oesophagus. Often you can feel the needle just under the skin on the right side, or you will see the feathers move as the needle passes beneath them.
12. Continue to only use two fingers and pass the gavage needle until the tip of the needle arrives at the crop. You may feel a small amount of resistance similar to pulling a glove over your fingers as the needle needs to push the oesophagus open as it passes down.
13. Gently inject the medication. If the volume is large enough, you will see the crop expand as it fills. Don't inject the solution too fast or the bird will regurgitate.
14. Once you have injected all the medication, slowly withdraw the needle, changing the angle as you leave the neck and pass into the mouth.
15. Continue to hold the bird quietly for approximately 30 seconds to give it a chance to adjust to the fluid in its crop.

Quick Summary of Important Points – where people usually go wrong

- Difficulty in passing the needle is usually due to holding the bird in an incorrect position. If the neck is not outstretched correctly, you cannot pass the needle easily. The neck must be stretched straight out, not kinked.
- Choose a large bore (diameter) needle – a small needle is more likely to enter the windpipe.
- Only use the strength of two fingers.
- Gently guide the needle down – don't push hard.
- Always pass the needle down the left-hand side of the mouth.
- Change the angle you guide the needle when you feel the needle tip leave the mouth.

- Don't inject the fluid quickly as this may result in stretching the crop and regurgitation.
- Don't put too large a volume into the crop. Use the table below as a guide.

Recommended Volume Administered into the Crop	
Species	**ml**
Finch	0.2
Canary	0.2
Budgerigar	0.5
Cockatiel	1.0
Small Parrot	2.0
Medium Parrot	5.0
Large Parrot	10.0

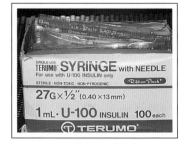

A syringe and needle combination useful for giving birds injections.

How to Give an Injection

From time to time you may need to give your bird an injection. In most cases this will be into the breast muscle. It is the largest muscle in the body and birds can absorb drugs from this site with amazing speed, certainly much more quickly than other animals.

Why bother? Well, if a bird is ill and you take the much easier option of placing the medication in its drinking water or food you may not properly medicate the bird. It is a well-known fact that ill birds eat and drink much less than normal. When we take medication, our doctor says: 'Take one tablet in the morning and another at night'. This allows us to have regular doses of the medicine and to take a known amount each time. When you place it in the water or food, you hope and pray that the bird takes enough in and at the right times. 'Murphy's Law' says that this usually will not happen. It is a common practice for many veterinarians to recommend an injection or a course of injections for a sick bird. If you are able to perform this deed at home, it may be less stressful on the patient.

Before you start, prepare the syringe and any equipment you will need. Lay it all out on a bench. Make sure that:
- All air bubbles have been removed from the syringe.
- You have the correct amount to inject in the syringe – if you are not certain, take the time to double check.
- You have a cottonwool ball ready and moistened with methylated spirits.

Take your bird in a comfortable hold so that you can easily reach the breast muscles

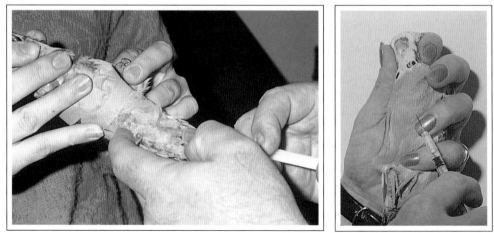

Left: Intramuscular injection.
Right: Giving an intramuscular injection into the large pectoral (breast) muscle.

and all the equipment you need is within easy reach. If you are nervous, sit down and make yourself relax. Make sure the bird is comfortable and is not struggling. If the bird is struggling a lot, it is usually a sign that it is being held incorrectly.

Use the index finger of your free hand to feel the keel bone running down the centre of the bird's breast. This is a very useful landmark. Take a ball of cottonwool that is moistened with methylated spirits and place it at the top of the keel bone. Run the cotton ball down towards the bird's vent. The feathers will be moistened and will part to reveal the keel bone and the muscle on either side. In all but very small birds, you should aim to inject at a site 0.5–1cm from the keel bone – usually in the middle of the breast muscle.

Hold the syringe between your thumb and index finger and aim the needle at 90 degrees to the skin. Push the needle in as far as it will go or until you feel resistance. Draw back on the plunger while looking at the hub of the needle. If blood comes into the needle hub, stop and withdraw the needle. If the needle hub is clear, inject the medication. The aim is to inject the medication as deeply as possible without injuring the patient. Gently withdraw the needle and apply pressure with your fingertip to stop any bleeding.

If giving a course of injections it is best to avoid injecting into the same site or you may damage the muscle at that site. To avoid this, I divide the breast muscle into four imaginary parts – upper right and left and lower right and left. I then always inject in a standard order.

Injection Number	Position
1	upper right
2	lower left
3	lower right
4	upper left

As most injections are not given more often than every 12 hours, this allows the bird to recover from each injection before the same site is reused.

BIRD RESTRAINT

Before any physical examination may be performed, it is necessary to catch and restrain the patient. In all cases this is different to the manner in which other animals are handled.

Handling and restraint of avian patients should:
1. Be safe and comfortable for the patient and handler.
2. Consider the behaviour of the bird.
3. Consider the physical characteristics of the bird.
4. Minimise stress.

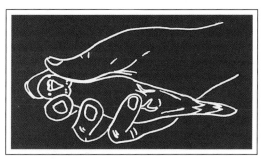

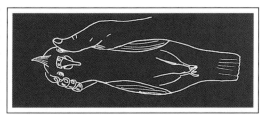

Drawings of how to hold small and large parrots. Note the position of the fingers. I prefer to use a towel as well to drape over the bird and the grip is applied over the towel. This means that they are not hand shy as it is the towel that 'grabbed' them.

Be Safe and Comfortable for the Patient and Handler

When performed for the first time in the presence of an owner, catching a bird can be a daunting and nerve-wracking experience. Take all precautions to make yourself comfortable. Sit down if it helps to relax you.

Avoid the temptation to use gloves with all birds (the only exception being raptors). As far as I am concerned, gloves have no place in restraining most cage birds, even with large cockatoos and macaws. Gloves reduce the sensitivity you have in feeling your patient and they are clumsy and awkward.

The preferred item for handling most aviary and pet birds is a towel. The thickness will vary with the size and biting power of the patient. I use tea-towels and face washers for most birds and a bath towel for large cockatoos. Towels are often unnecessary for handtamed pet birds. In many cases a towel has been used to tame the bird and is used in games. Take extra care using a towel with these birds to avoid making them fearful of what previously was fun. With these birds the towel should be slowly introduced from below and used to gently cuddle the bird. Many birds become docile in the dark interior of the towel and will still enjoy the towel game later.

In some birds the beak may be a potential cause of damage. Some people prefer to tape the beak closed to avoid this. I find this is usually unnecessary.

Consider the Behaviour of the Bird

The age of the bird will determine how it may respond to capture. Young birds may not have learned to be fearful of people. Older birds may have been caught many times and be aware of means to make the task more difficult. Aged birds may be at higher risk of diseases that may compromise capture.

Breeding status may complicate the issue. Birds that are handled and are incubating or feeding young may abandon the nest if captured and handled.

Health status is always a consideration. Any ill bird, particularly with respiratory disease, may be a poor candidate for capture and any handling must be kept to a minimum and avoided if possible.

The species of the patient may be a guide to handling. Large species such as Ostrich may require a shield to protect you as you push them along a race. Aggressive species such as cockatoos and lorikeets may attack you and fight. Other species, such as quail, may panic and erupt in flight crashing into walls or the roof, often with enough impact to cause serious damage or death.

Observe the bird to determine which methods of escape or defence it is likely to use.

Consider the Physical Characteristics of the Bird

An inspection of the bird's anatomy prior to attempting capture will make you aware of which structures it may use to defend itself, be it beak, wings, claws or legs.

The anatomy of birds makes capture a problem. They have air sacs and lack a diaphragm which makes them prone to problems if their chest movements are restricted. In long-necked birds, such as swans, excessive flexing of the neck or pressure, may kink or cause collapse of the trachea.

The bones of birds are fragile compared to mammals. They have thinner bones and some of the larger bones are pneumatic (air-filled).

Minimise Stress

Diurnal species are best caught in dim light or darkness. For nocturnal species the opposite applies. I find it useful to draw the curtains and make the room as dark as possible. I open the door and place my hand at the entrance. Once the bird settles down, I have an assistant (often the owner) switch the light off. The bird will usually freeze and can be quickly caught. Once the light comes back on, the bird is out of the cage with a minimum of fuss.

Before you attempt to restrain a bird have all your equipment prepared for any tests or medications you suspect you may need. This ensures that the bird is restrained for the minimum time possible.

To minimise any injuries, remove perches and other toys from the cage before you start the capture process. Make certain all doors and windows are closed prior to beginning the process.

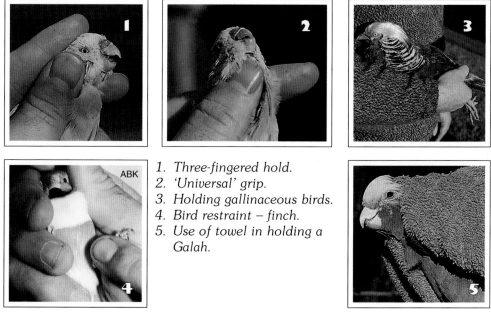

1. Three-fingered hold.
2. 'Universal' grip.
3. Holding gallinaceous birds.
4. Bird restraint – finch.
5. Use of towel in holding a Galah.

Capture Technique

Approach the bird from behind. This is not as important if you intend to simply throw a towel over the bird. Aim to grasp the head and upper surface of the body, including the wings, and gently press the bird onto the wall or floor.

If a towel is used, gently remove the whole bundle from the cage usually with pressure only maintained around the head and neck. This is useful if you have to catch the bird in a small cage and remove it through a small opening. Simply allow the cloth to fold over the bird and then pull the bundle through the opening. Once the bird is removed from the cage adjust your grip and restrain the feet if necessary. The towel may be kept around the bird or removed as the situation indicates.

Release

This should occur as soon as possible. Birds should not be restrained for long periods. Turn the bird to the correct orientation. I like to release them onto the ground so that they can adjust to new bearings and are less likely to panic or flutter. For large and aggressive species I give them a gentle push so that they don't turn around and attack. Above all, do not release birds in midair. This is dangerous and stressful for the patient.

Holding the Patient

The grip you use is often a matter of personal preference. Despite the grip used, the position of the fingers is of utmost importance. As birds lack a diaphragm, they use movement of the sternum to move air through their air sacs and lungs. If you encircle the bird's body with your fingers you will interfere with the bird's breathing movements and cause asphyxiation. Many birds have died simply from incorrect handling.

Parrots

I find that if the head is correctly held with the correct amount of tension and the neck is stretched and extended, most birds will lie quietly. For small to medium sized birds, my preference is for the three-finger hold. This triangulation of fingers holds the head still and does not put pressure on the chest. For larger parrots I use a grip with the heel of the thumb on one side and all my fingers on the other side. The remainder of the parrot is covered by a towel or by my other hand gripping the wing tips, tail and feet.

An alternative grip is used by some practitioners. Termed the 'Universal' grip, it can be used for all parrots from Budgerigars to large cockatoos. The thumb is inserted into the gap underneath the lower beak. The index finger encircles the back of the neck placing a downward pressure on both of the wings. This allows the neck to be extended. This requires more skill to master but can be a very useful technique.

Passerines

Canaries and finches can be restrained by the three-finger method or simply held with their neck between the index and second finger as the other fingers lightly enclose the wings and feet.

Pigeons

Racing pigeons are held in the palm, facing towards you. The feet are held between the index and second finger while the tail and wing tips are encircled by the thumb. Native pigeons may panic when held like this. Hold small species like passerines. The hand is placed over the back of the bird with the bird's head falling between the index finger and the third finger. These two fingers are folded under to support the breast. The remaining fingers and thumb lightly support the body and enclose the wings. Some of the larger species are remarkably strong and are able to push themselves free with their wings if held loosely. Using both hands and with the bird facing away from you, the thumbs are placed along the bird's back. The remaining fingers are folded around the bird's body and the base of the palm is used to enclose the wings. The head and neck rest on the finger tips.

Gallinaceous Birds

Pheasants, poultry etc are held with the head between my chest wall and upper arm. The feet are held by one hand with the index finger separating them. In this position the vent is facing away from you and no nasty deposits end up in your pocket. Small species such as quail may be held as for passerines.

Raptors

Hawks, eagles etc are handled with gloves. They may be restrained with hood, jesses, swivels and leashes as commonly used for falconry. Alternately, they may be held in one or two hands with the wing tips and tail encircled and the feet separated by the fingers.

Wild Birds

A modification of the above techniques may be selected depending on the bird's size and shape.

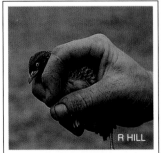

*Single-handed
handling Quail*

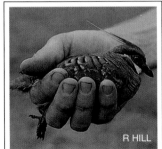

*Single-handed
handling Pigeons*

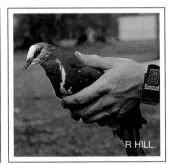

*Double-handed
handling Pigeons*

COMMON PROBLEMS

When you gather a list of common problems it is often enough to worry people that birds appear to have a lot of diseases. Do not let this list alarm you. As a general rule, most birds are quite healthy.

This list should help you to detect the early signs of disease and work with your veterinarian to begin treatment early on in the disease process. Use this list as a guide to monitor your birds particularly when purchasing new stock and during the quarantine period after you bring them home.

Because they often live very closely with their owner, many birds are exposed to psychological stress. Nearly all parrots are intelligent birds and when handreared and kept with people, they rely on them for their emotional needs. Often we do not meet their needs as well as we should. It takes some imagination and commitment to make these pet birds as happy as they should be.

When you do have disease problems always be critical of your management techniques. Try to find some management changes that will avoid the problem in the future. Be particularly aware of the role stress plays in weakening an animal which allows diseases, that it would normally be able to fight, to get out of control. The times when birds are more prone to the effects of stress are during moulting, breeding or when moved to a new home.

If your bird is ill always ask yourself: 'Is there something I have done that may have stressed the bird to allow this to occur?' Even when an infectious disease is the cause of the illness, it may be stress that has allowed the problem to arise.

INFECTIOUS DISEASES

Mycoplasmosis
Signs:
- Swelling around the eyes.
- Sneezing.
- Nasal discharge.

This is an upper respiratory infection caused by small organisms called *Mycoplasma*. Often it will cause disease in combination with *Chlamydophila psittaci* or a virus. It can be quite contagious. Ill birds should be isolated as far from the other birds as possible. There are records of this being passed from Budgerigars to Cockatiels, so it is best to avoid mixing these species in an aviary.

Treatment usually requires a course of antibiotics such as Tylosin™, Spectinomycin™ or Baytril™. These may be given by injection, in drinking water or some birds may require a nebuliser. Treatment is usually needed for any other infections that may be present. As well, you need to identify the cause of any stress present and remove it.

Intestinal Worms
Signs:
- Weight loss.
- Depression.
- Diarrhoea.

Worms are still a common problem in birds. The most likely worm to be found in Australian parrots is the roundworm. This is passed on by birds coming into contact with their own droppings, or droppings from other birds, that contain the worm eggs. To avoid this it is recommended that you remove the build-up of droppings on the floor of their cage as often as possible. A minimum would be once a week. Use concrete or wire floors to aid hygiene. If problems arise with worms such as gizzardworm or tapeworm, it is recommended to use an insecticide such as Coopex™, to control the insects that carry these worms.

If large numbers of worms build up in the intestine they can cause a blockage that will result in death. Worm problems will occur when the hygiene in the aviary is not as good as it should be or when there are high levels of humidity. It can also be a problem for laying hens as they are confined to a small space in the nest and it is a stressful time for them.

It is recommended that you give your birds a worm treatment after each breeding round or at times of high humidity and stress. Most of the drugs used are not registered for use in birds so you must assume responsibility for their use. (For detailed account and preventative treatments refer to *Avian Parasite Control* on page 86).

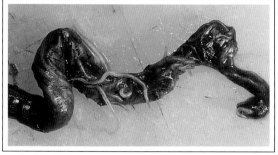

Chlamydophilosis (Psittacosis)

Signs:
- Poor looking bird.
- Ruffled feathers/huddled posture.
- Depression.
- Weight loss.
- Conjunctivitis.
- Feather loss around one or both eyes.
- Sinusitis.
- Nostrils plugged.
- Sneezing.
- Heavy breathing (tail bobbing).
- Soiled vent.
- Diarrhoea – often a lime-green colour.
- Excessive urine in droppings.
- Sudden death.

Above: Multiple roundworms in the intestine of a Northern Rosella.
Below: Capillaria – hairworm or wireworm that irritates the intestine and can lead to death.

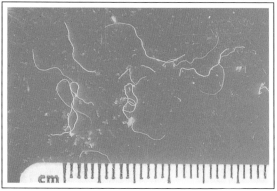

This is a very common infectious disease. A large number of birds carry the *Chlamydophila psittaci* organism in their system but will only show signs of disease when stressed. Some birds are carriers and will shed the organism to infect other birds but not show signs themselves. There are laboratory tests your veterinarian can perform to detect the organism in your bird. Birds that survive infection are often still fully susceptible to the disease.

Treatment is a long drawn out process. The drug of choice is doxycycline (Psittavet™). It can be administered by injections once a week or as drinking water medication. The birds must be treated for a minimum of six weeks. If they are treated for a lesser time, they will look fine for a while but then develop signs again, when they relapse.

This disease is of particular concern as it can also be passed on to people. The symptoms are often like a cold or flu that won't clear up. It can cause severe illness in people. If at any time, you are ill it is important to mention to your doctor that you have birds at home. (For a more detailed account refer to *Psittacosis* on page 96).

Candidiasis

Signs:
- Vomiting and regurgitation.
- White plaques in the mouth.
- Crop may feel thickened.

- Slowed crop emptying in nestlings/handreared birds.
- Diarrhoea – with sweet odour.

This is a disease that is caused by a yeast, *Candida albicans,* which mainly affects the mouth and crop. It is more common in young birds, particularly if they are handreared. The yeast is common around people and can be contained in our saliva or on our hands. It is important that you do not allow saliva to come into contact with the bird's food. Hands should be always washed well before handling birds and a general high level of hygiene maintained.

Antibiotics that kill yeasts must be used. In most cases nystatin (Nilstat™ or Mycostatin™) given at 0.25–0.5ml three times daily is successful. In some cases the yeasts will be resistant and other drugs such as ketoconazole (Nizoral™) are required. Treatment is maintained until 2–3 days after all signs have gone. Aviclens™ in the drinking water, 5ml per 10 litres of water, also has a yeast inhibitory action and will help to decrease the amount passed between birds.

Giardiasis
Signs:
- Weight loss.
- Excessive feather grooming.
- Oily, greasy feathers.
- Feather picking and screaming.
- Whole seeds in droppings.
- Diarrhoea.
- Enlarged droppings
  (stool component).
- Deaths in young birds.

This disease is caused by a protozoan parasite, *Giardia lamblia.* It is common in the USA but not in Australia. It is present in the drinking water of many of the cities in Australia and there are suspicions that it may increase as a cause of problems in both birds and people in the future.

It can be a difficult organism to detect and is often not seen until post-mortem examination. It is possible to test the bird's droppings but they must be very fresh, preferably still warm, as the organisms die when the droppings cool down.

Treatment is with Emtryl™ or Ronivet-S™ at the dose recommended by the manufacturer. Flagyl Suspension™ (200mg/ml), 3.5ml per litre of water, or Torgyl Solution™ (5mg/ml), 2ml per litre of water, have also been used alone or in combination with Emtryl™ or Ronivet-S™.

Kidney Infections/Tumours
Signs:
- Lethargy and depression.
- Weight loss.
- Enlarged abdomen.
- Wet droppings.
- Lameness in one leg (occasionally two legs).

Problems with the kidney are quite common in birds. This is because the blood flow from the legs and feet can be naturally diverted to flow through the kidney where it acts as a filter to trap infection. In a normal bird, this is not a problem, but in a bird with disease in the leg or foot this can lead to kidney infection or damage. One of the most common signs of kidney disease is excess fluid in the droppings.

In some birds, damage to the kidney causes the kidney to swell. This can place pressure on the sciatic nerve which passes through the kidney and the bird will show as lame. It will rest the upper part of its leg on the perch as it cannot grip with its foot. This form of lameness can be seen with kidney infection as well as a tumour (cancer) of either the kidney or the gonad (testis or ovary) as in both these situations there will be pressure on the sciatic nerve. The birds that most commonly have kidney tumours are Budgerigars, in most other birds, infection or poisoning are the most common causes of these signs.

All birds with kidney disease need fluid therapy (see *Fluid Therapy – Electrolytes* on page 20). Other treatments will depend upon the cause. If an infection is suspected, antibiotics will be needed. For gout, allopurinol (Zyloprim™) is used; for tumours, no treatment will be successful as they are usually too large to be removed surgically, so the emphasis is on making the bird comfortable and considering euthanasia when it becomes too ill.

Bacterial Infections
Signs:
- Poor looking bird.
- Ruffled feathers/huddled posture.
- Depression.
- Weight loss.
- Conjunctivitis.
- Feather loss around one or both eyes.
- Sinusitis.
- Nostrils plugged.
- Sneezing.
- Heavy breathing (tail bobbing).
- Soiled vent.
- Diarrhoea – often a lime-green colour.
- Excessive urine in droppings.
- Sudden death.

There are a very large number of bacteria that can cause disease in birds. The most common ones cause a septicaemia where the poisons from the bacteria make the bird look generally ill. The signs may be indistinguishable from Chlamydophilosis.

As a general rule, all bacteria can be divided into two groups based on laboratory tests using a Gram stain – Gram positive and Gram negative. In most cases it is the Gram negative bacteria that cause problems in birds. These are a diverse group and the antibiotic that is best for them can vary. Often your veterinarian will begin the bird on an antibiotic and then send a swab away to a laboratory to culture (grow and identify) the bacteria and to perform a sensitivity test. This tests the bacteria against a range of antibiotics to help choose the best one to use.

Spirochaetes have been found in Cockatiels to cause a disease similar to a cold or flu. The birds are depressed and sneeze. Doxycycline at the dose used for *Chlamydophila psittaci* should be a successful treatment.

Respiratory Infections
Problems in the respiratory system are quite common in birds. The problems can be divided into two basic groups.
1. Those affecting the upper respiratory tract (nose, sinuses and windpipe) or
2. Those affecting the lower respiratory tract (air sacs and lungs).

It is common for the disease to begin in the upper airways and then spread to the lower airways.

Upper Airway Disease (nose, sinuses and windpipe)
Signs:
- Staining of feathers above the nostrils.
- Swelling around the eyes or corner of the mouth.
- Blockage of the nostrils.

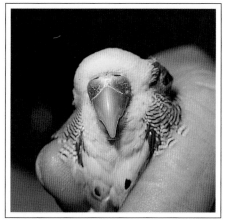

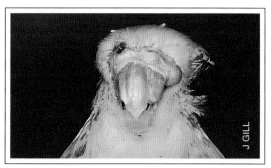

Left: This is often mistaken for eye problems but is actually an infection in the sinus. Eye ointment is a waste of time. This bird needs antibiotic injections.
Below: Severe upper respiratory infection. This bird was not treated with injections and the sinus infection became much worse.

- Open-mouth breathing.
- Noisy breathing.
- Sneezing.

This is a particularly common problem in many parrots and pigeons. The most common problem is Upper Respiratory Tract Infection (URTI). In many cases this is associated with *Chlamydophila psittaci* (Psittacosis), *Mycoplasma* or a range of bacteria. Vitamin A deficiency may also play a role.

The swelling around the eye is a problem that is often mistaken as an eye disease. It actually is a problem in the bird's sinuses and will not improve with eye ointment. The majority of these birds need an injectable antibiotic (doxycycline or enrofloxacin are the best choices).

Some birds will need eye surgery to remove the build-up of pus that occurs in the sinus. If the pus is not removed, the problem will settle down and then recur later. In-water medication is only useful in these birds if you catch them in the early stages of the disease.

Allergies in birds can occur but are not common. Some birds are allergic to cigarette smoke and will have recurring problems if kept enclosed in a household with heavy smokers in the family.

Irritation from fumes can be a problem. The most common causes are build-up of dust, ammonia from the urates and household chemicals (insecticides, disinfectants etc).

Lower Airway Disease (air sacs and lungs)
Signs:
- Tail bobbing.
- Open-mouth breathing.
- Noisy breathing.
- Loss of voice/song.
- Loss of appetite.
- Poor flying (weakness).

These birds usually have very fast and laboured breathing. They sit hunched on the perch and are bobbing their tail to help with breathing. In advanced cases they breathe through their mouth and have their neck stretched out. If you hold the bird close to your ear you can hear wheezing, whistling or gurgling sounds.

In most cases this develops into a generalised disease involving the lower airways and the rest of the body. This is usually associated with *Chlamydophila psittaci* (Psittacosis), *Mycoplasma* or a range of bacteria. Vitamin A deficiency may also play a role. Outside Australia, *Mycobacterium* (Tuberculosis) is a major problem. In some species (Budgerigars, penguins, pigeons, magpies, waterfowl and Cockatiels),

Aspergillus (a fungus that grows in the air sacs) may be a major problem.

Mycoplasma is the cause of the 'one-eyed cold'. It usually responds to tylosin (Tylan™) or tiamulin (Dynamutalin™).

Sunken Eye Syndrome

Signs:

- Sinus infection followed by the eye sinking.

This disease has not been reported in Australia. The problem begins with an infection in the bird's sinus (around the eyes). It is usually associated with Gram negative bacteria and so will respond to antibiotic injections. Often a culture and sensitivity test will need to be done to confirm the best antibiotic. Once the infection is cured, the eye usually returns to its normal position.

It has been found in Yellow-collared Macaws, Scarlet Macaws and Green-winged Macaws, conures and Emus.

Megabacteria (Avian Gastric Yeast)

Signs:

- Weight loss over variable periods up to 18 months.
- Increased appetite.
- Occasional vomiting.
- Frothy droppings.
- Undigested food in faeces.
- Bulky, soft faeces.
- Blood in faeces.
- Black, tarry faeces.

This disease is caused by an organism that has been identified as a yeast or fungus, so it is not really a type of bacteria. This means that we now have a path to investigate new treatments. Research is still being done to classify it fully. It is primarily seen in the Budgerigar but may occasionally be seen in poultry, canaries, Peachfaced Lovebirds, Cockatiels, Neophema Grass Parrots and other parrots. It is important to note that birds vary in susceptibility to this disease. The disease may be present in an aviary but only some of the birds will have problems.

Diagnosis is based on detecting the organisms in the droppings, although this can be unreliable. The most reliable means is to detect the organism at post-mortem. It is hoped that, in time, new and better tests will become available so that carrier birds can be identified and removed from the breeding birds. Contact your veterinarian about these tests.

Treatment has variable success. Most commonly used treatments are Fungilin Suspension™ as drops to the mouth or Fungilin Lozenges™ dissolved in drinking water. The water soluble Megabac-S™ is another alternative. Treatment needs to be for a minimum of two weeks. Relapses occur commonly. Research is being done to identify new medications to help with this disease.

Trichomoniasis

Signs:

- White, cheesy material in the mouth or throat.
- Vomiting seed or crop contents.
- Dry retching or neck stretching.
- Green diarrhoea.
- Loose droppings (mostly urates with no faeces).
- Birds may be depressed and listless.
- Weight loss.
- Death.

This disease has been recognised for a long time. In raptors it is called 'frounce'. In

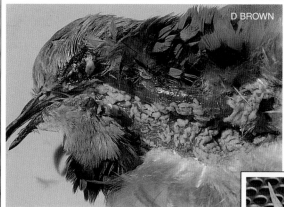

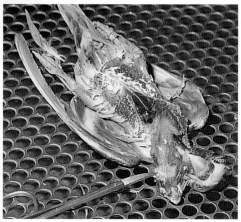

Left: Trichomoniasis (Canker) in pigeon.
Below: Trichomoniasis. The white scarring which the scissors are pointing to, is due to a protozoan infection. The extent of scarring stopped the bird being able to swallow properly.

many other birds it is called 'canker' or 'trich'.

The cause of this problem is a very small protozoan called *Trichomonas gallinae*. It can affect the bird in any area from the mouth to the crop and oesophagus. The organism burrows into the tissue lining and causes a large white, cheesy reaction. If left untreated 50% of birds will die.

The scarring that occurs with chronic Trichomoniasis, usually blocks the passage of food down the oesophagus. The birds will be seen sitting constantly at the food bowl and appear to be eating. In fact, they cannot swallow the seed and are slowly starving. A characteristic sign in Budgerigars is vomiting large amounts of mucous while throwing their head around. The mucous is thrown back onto their head and then dries causing the feathers around the face to be plastered down. They look like an escapee from a Brylcreem™ commercial.

The disease is passed on by a bird eating food, or drinking water, that has been contaminated by vomit or saliva from an infected bird. In aviaries it is very contagious. Similarly, it can be passed from parent to a young chick during the feeding in the nest. Not all birds with this organism look ill. Some look absolutely normal and act as carriers, to infect other birds around them.

Diagnosis is by examining a 'crop wash' from a live bird. In a dead bird the typical white, cheesy material will be seen at post-mortem examination. Conditions that mimic this problem include Vitamin A deficiency, Poxvirus, Candidiasis, food caught in the mouth or burns to the lining of the mouth from disinfectants that have not been diluted properly.

To prevent the problem entering your bird collection, I would recommend treating all new Budgerigars and pigeons during the quarantine period, before they are placed in with your other birds.

Effective disinfectants for use in an aviary or cage are: Iodines, Quaternary Ammonium compounds or Chlorhexidine.

Effective treatments are ronidazole (Ronivet™, Turbosole™), dimetridazole (Emtryl™), metronidazole (Flagyl™, Torgyl™, Metrin™) or carnidazole (Spartrix™).

Birds that have problems with Trichomoniasis include Budgerigars, pigeons, doves, quail, raptors and canaries.

Scaly-face Mite

Signs:
- Crusts on unfeathered parts of the face (eyelids, around the beak).
- Honeycomb appearance to these white crusty masses.

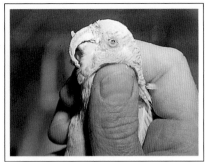

Scaly-face Mite in Budgerigar causing deformed beak.

The mite causes a build-up of crusty material as a response to the irritation it causes.

In parrots, it most commonly is found around the face but it can also be on the skin of the preen gland, vent, legs and feet. In severe cases, it will be on the skin between the rows of feathers on the wings.

In passerines, such as the canary, the crusting is most commonly found on the legs and feet. It causes large thin crusts to grow out from the bottom of the feet. The common name for this is 'tassle foot'.

This condition can be confused with other causes of thickening of the skin. Canaries and finches may have thickening of the skin covering the feet due to malnutrition or old age. The condition could also be due to Poxvirus infection or dried food on the beak.

Bird species which have this problem include Budgerigars, Neophemas (especially Scarlet-chested Parrots), Kakarikis, Princess Parrots, canaries and the European Goldfinch.

Coccidiosis

Signs:
- Diarrhoea (sometimes with blood present).
- Weight loss.
- Dehydration.
- Birds are depressed and listless.
- Sudden death.

The *Coccidia* are protozoan parasites that live in the lining of the bird's intestine. They damage the intestine and may cause haemorrhage. Birds are unable to absorb nutrients from their food. This can eventually lead to death.

The Coccidiosis is passed between birds by eating another bird's droppings containing the *Coccidia* 'eggs'. These eggs, passed in the droppings, are quite small and are called oocysts. Diagnosis is by examining the droppings under a microscope and identifying the oocysts.

Large numbers of oocysts can be passed in the droppings and contaminate an aviary very quickly. The problem is very contagious and many deaths can suddenly occur. Poor hygiene and overcrowded aviaries are a common cause of outbreaks. When a bird only has low levels of infection, it may not show any symptoms. Canaries with Coccidiosis may be described as having 'black spot'. This is a large dark area under the skin of the abdomen and is caused by the liver being enlarged. This is a special type of *Coccidia* called *Atoxoplasma*.

Treatment for Coccidiosis is usually by adding coccidiostats to the drinking water. Common examples are toltrazuril (Baycox™), amprolium (Amprolmix Plus™ or Coccivet™) and sulfa drugs (eg Tribrissen Water Medication™, Sulpha D™ or Sulpha 3™).

Birds that have problems with Coccidiosis include canaries, finches, waterfowl, quail, Budgerigars, pigeons and poultry.

Lice

Signs:
- Excessive chewing or preening of feathers/skin.
- Bald spots.

- Damaged feathers.
- Presence of lice or eggs on plumage.

Most lice will go onto any bird. As a general rule they are more common on passerines and pigeons than parrots.

To check a bird for lice, spread the wing out and hold it up to a strong light. The lice can be seen moving along the feathers. The eggs are small dark spots near the feather shaft.

The lice cannot live for very long away from the bird. Control is aimed at using 'safe' insecticides on the bird. Treatments include dusting with Carbaryl™ or pyrethrin powders or sprays, once a week until all lice are removed or ivermectin or moxidectin drops into the mouth or onto the skin on the back of the neck once weekly until all lice are removed. This normally requires only 2–3 treatments to clear a bird.

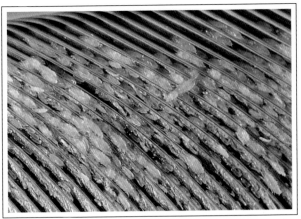

Close-up view of a heavy lice burden in the feather barbs of a Budgerigar.

Air Sac Mite

Signs:
- Heavy breathing.
- Open-mouth breathing.
- Stain on feathers around nostrils.
- Coughing (clicking sounds).
- Sneezing.
- Birds stop singing.

These are small, dark mites that are found in the windpipe and air sacs. They cause irritation and eventually lead to asphyxiation. It is thought they spread from adults to young birds when they are being fed.

The birds will have a wheezing or whistle to their breathing when held up to your ear. The most effective treatment is ivermectin or moxidectin as drops into the mouth (See *Common Parasiticides* on page 91). Shelltox Pest Strips™, at a rate of 1 strip per 10 cubic metres, placed in the aviary where birds cannot come into contact with the strip, have also been used by some aviculturists as a control mechanism. Take care using these strips. They contain a strong poison and if the birds drink from the moisture beads that form on the strip or drop to the ground, they may die.

Bird species which have this problem include the Gouldian Finch, Cordon Bleu Finch, European Goldfinch and the canary in Australia. Overseas it is also reported in parakeets and Cockatiels.

Toe Constriction Syndrome

Signs:
- Circular constriction around the toe.
- Loss of toes.

This is occasionally seen as a tightening of a band around one or more toes. Eventually it constricts the toe and the blood supply is blocked. The toe initially swells then shrivels up, dies and eventually drops off.

The cause is not certain but theories include trauma and low humidity problems (below 50% – especially in the brooder).

Treatment, in the early stages, is surgery to remove the constriction, as well as poultices, warm water soaks and massage to help restore blood flow and save the toe. Some people have had success with massaging an ointment containing tetracycline (Latycin™ or Terramycin™) into the area. Dimethyl sulphoxide (DMSO) paint has been used to reduce inflammation. In advanced stages the toe may need to be amputated. It is occasionally seen in Eclectus Parrots, African Grey Parrots and macaws, particularly in very young birds.

Viral Diseases
Circovirus
(Psittacine Beak and
Feather Disease)
Signs:

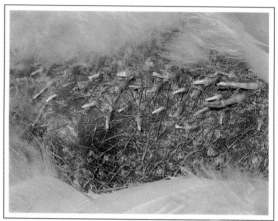

- More common in young birds, usually under one year of age.
- Abnormal feather growth particularly primary flight and crest feathers.
- Loss of powder down feathers.
- Shiny beak in cockatoos.
- Dirty plumage.
- Patches of yellow feathers appear in a green bird or white feathers in a blue bird.
- Bald patches anywhere on the body.
- Does not affect the beak in most parrots other than cockatoos.
- Secondary infections.
- Sneezing.
- Conjunctivitis.
- Diarrhoea.
- Excess or abnormal urine/urates.

Close-up of powder down feathers in the hip region of a Sulphur-crested Cockatoo with Psittacine Beak and Feather Disease. Note the feathers (which normally look like a very fluffy feather duster) are small, twisted and deformed. This is often the first sign that the bird has this disease.

This disease has been found in Australia, North America, Europe and Asia. The virus

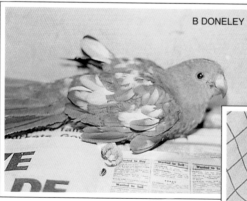

B DONELEY

is found in feather dust and any discharge (saliva, tears, droppings, crop contents) shed by infected birds. Cleaning the bird's environment regularly to minimise dust present is a useful tool in reducing the amount of viral particles that can be passed to

Above: Yellow feathers in King Parrot with PBFD.
Right: Blue Princess Parrot with PBFD.
(Note patches of white feathers.)

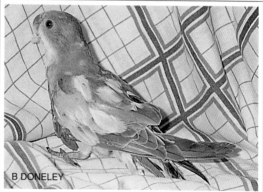

B DONELEY

other birds. The viral particles in dust can be passed around an aviary by natural airflow or on footwear, clothing, nets, carry cages, food and water dishes or vermin. Laboratory tests can help identify infected birds, which should be isolated from any other birds, particularly breeding birds. As the virus is present in wild parrots in Australia, they can be a source of passing the virus. Use solid roofing and walls in the construction of your aviary to restrict access for wild birds.

Circovirus causes Psittacine Beak and Feather Disease (PBFD). It is most common in cockatoos but may occasionally cause problems in other parrots. Blood tests and examination of feathers will help detect this virus.

There is no treatment available, however, vaccination should be available very soon. If the bird is close to breeding birds, it should be removed and isolated. If the bird has reached the stage where secondary illnesses are making it ill, euthanasia should be considered.

Polyomavirus (Papovavirus)
Signs:
In young birds
- Enlarged abdomen.
- Crop emptying slowly or not at all.
- Bruising under the skin.
- Death within 2–3 days.
In older birds
- Abnormal flight and tail feathers.
- Weight loss.
- Poor growth.

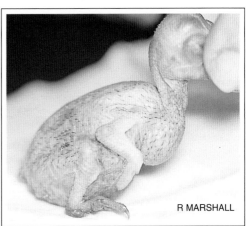
R MARSHALL

Polyomavirus in Eclectus chick.

This virus has been found worldwide in parrots, finches and gallinaceous birds (eg pheasants, chickens, turkeys and waterfowl).

This is a cause of death in young birds that have not fledged. It can affect both parent raised or handreared birds. This virus can be carried by the adult birds with no signs shown at all. In adult Eclectus Parrots it can cause illness and death. It is more common in aviaries that use multiple clutches and an all-year breeding cycle. Strict hygiene is necessary where any birds are being handreared as it is very contagious and easily passed on by the people handling the birds.

There is no treatment for this disease. In a breeding situation the best control measure is to cease breeding for up to one year.

Glutaraldehyde is a disinfectant (refer to *Disinfection* on page 100). This is effective to use in cleaning the environment and any utensils. A thorough cleaning and removal of all biological material (droppings, feathers, food etc), prior to applying the disinfectant, is essential.

Disease Prevention in an Aviary
(How do I stop the Polyomavirus entering my aviary?)
- If you breed parrots, do not breed Budgerigars, lovebirds or Cockatiels on the premises unless each individual has had its blood tested for Polyomavirus.
- Raise your own young. Do not bring babies from another aviary onto the premises.
- If a bird leaves the aviary (eg for a bird show or on breeding loan), and then returns, it should be quarantined and have its blood tested before being used for breeding or mixing with the aviary birds.
- Any new bird entering the aviary should test negative for Polyomavirus before mixing with breeding birds.
- The most common cause of transmitting a virus is through people (on hands, clothes,

shoes etc). Control people moving around the aviary. They should move from the birds most likely to be infected and progress towards the least likely to be infected but more likely to be a carrier. This makes it less likely that the virus can move toward the birds with the highest risk of infection.

- Visitors (bird dealers, delivery trucks and other aviculturists) should not visit areas where there are breeding birds or nestlings.
- If you show birds, they should be housed in a separate building and remain separated from the breeding establishment until the end of the season. Any birds intended for breeding at the end of the season should test negative for Polyomavirus before entering the breeding group.
- Do not introduce birds under 18 weeks of age into the aviary. Make sure that all birds introduced into the aviary are fully weaned.

Disease Control in an Aviary
(What do I do if I have a Polyomavirus outbreak?)
- Once you have the virus identified (by a post-mortem examination and laboratory tests on a sick bird), be aware that little can be done for any exposed nestlings; most will succumb to the virus.
- Look at the hygiene in the aviary and make any improvements you can.
- Do not move any birds.
- Control people moving around the aviary. They should move from the birds most likely to be infected and progress towards the least likely to be infected but more likely to be a carrier. This makes it less likely the virus can move toward the birds with the highest risk of infection.
  - Do not allow any visitors to enter your aviaries. Do not visit other aviaries.
  - Only regular aviary staff should move around the aviary.
  - Do not take any birds to a show. You will not cause a problem in older birds, but they can act as carriers and transport the virus to their establishment.
  - Stop breeding birds.
  - Do not handrear any birds. Leave them in the nest to be parent reared. Parent raised chicks (except in Budgerigars and lovebirds) are more resistant to the virus.
- After the outbreak has stopped, inspect the aviary thoroughly and identify possible birds which introduced the virus. These should be blood tested and/or removed from the aviary. Do a thorough cleaning and disinfection of the aviary and nursery.
- The virus is maintained in the aviary by shedding from infected nestlings and juvenile or sub-adult birds. To break the cycle you need to stop breeding for 6–12 months and remove all young birds. Regularly disinfect the aviary over the 6–12 months. It is usually safe to begin breeding again as long as all carrier birds have been identified by blood tests and eliminated.
- Use the strategies listed under *Disease Prevention in an Aviary* to stop the virus entering again.

Pacheco's Disease Virus
Signs:
- Sudden death.
- Depression.
- Ruffled feathers.
- Diarrhoea (yellow-green).
- Excess urine.
- Excessive drinking.
- Death within a few days.

This is an acute disease caused by a Herpesvirus. Diagnosis is usually based upon finding at post-mortem examination and samples sent to a pathologist for testing.

Patagonian and Nanday Conures are regarded as carriers of this virus, so they should be held separately from other parrots.

There is no treatment, but eight capsules of acyclovir (Zovirax™, 200mg capsules) per 4.5 litres of drinking water for 14 days, have had some success in controlling outbreaks. This helps to protect birds that have not contracted the virus. If the birds are already incubating the virus, even if no signs are yet evident, the disease will progress as normal.

As an alternative, Aviclens™ added to the water can help kill the virus and slow down the spread of the infection. It can also be used for disinfecting the premises and utensils. Do not use Aviclens™ and Zovirax™ in the water together.

Management procedures are aimed at reducing the birds' exposure to faeces from other birds, as the virus is passed out in the faeces. Remove and replace the paper at the bottom of the cage at least once a day. Wash your hands regularly in Hibiclens™ disinfectant. House birds separately or in numbers that avoid overcrowding.

Proventricular Dilatation Disease (PDD)

This disease was first reported in the 1970s. The cause is unknown, but a virus is suspected. It appears to be contagious, with birds developing symptoms between four and eight months after being exposed to a sick bird.

Initially it was only seen in macaws (particularly Blue and Gold and Green-winged Macaws) but has since been seen in many parrot species such as African Grey Parrots, Amazons, Cockatiels, cockatoos, conures,

Enlarged proventriculus (the white area) of a Military Macaw. It died after showing symptoms of PDD – weight loss and undigested seed in the faeces.

Eclectus, macaws, Senegals and Thick-billed Parrots.

Only one case has been reported in Australia in a young macaw. This was a bird that had been recently imported from overseas. No other cases have been reported in Australia, even in birds that had close contact with this bird.

Often the first sign is vomiting or regurgitation. This is followed by depression, weight loss and a poor appetite. Often undigested seed will be passed in the droppings. The birds are quite weak and will often have diarrhoea and excessive urine in their droppings. Some birds can be kept alive on liquid diets for some time but all birds, with this disease, eventually die.

This problem should be suspected in macaws that are weaned and growing well, who revert to begging to be handfed.

Often it is a difficult disease to diagnose with 100% accuracy. There are many diseases that mimic the signs seen with this disease, such as any infections or obstructions in the gizzard or proventriculus, heavy metal poisoning, Megabacteria infection in the proventriculus, Vitamin E deficiency or intestinal Papillomatosis.

The most reliable test to confirm this disease is a biopsy of the gizzard. More recently biopsy samples are being taken from the lining of the crop, as it is simpler surgery. Unfortunately biopsies are not 100% accurate.

Other tests that help with diagnosis are an X-ray or endoscopy to help detect the swollen proventriculus that is seen with this disease. Unfortunately, because there are other causes of a swollen proventriculus, these tests are also not 100% accurate in diagnosing PDD.

Because PDD is such a difficult disease to diagnose, it is most commonly diagnosed from samples collected during the post-mortem examination and sent to a pathologist. Other names for the same disease are: Macaw Wasting Syndrome, Macaw Fading Syndrome, Gastric Distension of Macaws, Myenteric Ganglioneuritis, Psittacine Wasting Disease, Proventricular Dilatation of Psittacines, Psittacine Proventricular Dilatation Syndrome (PPDS).

Psittacine Pruritic Polyfolliculosis

This is a name for a disease syndrome that is found in Budgerigars and African Lovebirds and occasionally other birds such as Galahs and Sulphur-crested Cockatoos. Initially it was called Budgerigar Short Tail Disease but this name has changed as it is a problem in birds other than Budgerigars, and not all birds have a short tail.

This disease is a form of self-mutilation where the birds appear to be very itchy on their rump, neck or shoulders. The birds appear to be intensely preening. They chew viciously at the affected areas and eventually cause damage to the skin so an ulcerated area is formed. If you look closely, you can see some feather follicles have more than one feather growing. This is because the initial feather has been damaged and now has the appearance of multiple feathers. In other sites, the feathers will be twisted and deformed or some feathers will be underneath the skin and twisted in a circle.

At the moment this is thought to be caused by a virus, but one has not yet been identified. In the past this problem has been called 'stress dermatitis' at other times a poxvirus has been suggested as the cause.

Diseases that can be confused with this one are: PBFD, Papovavirus infection or infections of the feather follicle with either *Chlamydophila psittaci* or bacteria.

To date no treatment has been completely successful. Some birds can be kept comfortable with depot injections of cortisone, combined with soothing lotions or Dimethyl sulphoxide (DMSO) paint. As well, I have had success with an Elizabethan Collar or neck brace to stop excessive chewing and the formation of scar tissue. Homeopathic treatments, using combinations of Australian bushflower essences, have shown some initial success at controlling symptoms, but not cure.

Nestling Viral Diseases

Because of their age and the fact that their immune system is not fully developed, juvenile birds are prone to infections by a number of viruses. These viruses may be passed to the young if the parents are carriers.

The two most common viral infections seen in juvenile parrots are:
Polyomavirus (Papovavirus)
Signs:
- Sudden onset of illness.
- Slow crop emptying.
- Listlessness.
- Vomiting.
- Blood spots on the skin.
- Sudden death.
- Abnormal feather growth.

Polyomavirus (Papovavirus) is quite common. It usually affects very young nestlings. Often the first sign you will see is a dead chick. Most birds will die within 48 hours of looking ill. Any birds that survive will grow more slowly than normal, be prone to developing secondary bacterial infections and may develop deformed feathers. These birds will mimic the feather loss seen with PBFD (*Circovirus*). In some cases the birds may develop deformity of the beak or legs.

Psittacine Beak and Feather Disease (PBFD)
Signs:
- Slow onset of illness.
- Weight loss.
- Listlessness.
- Begging to be fed.
- Loss of powder down (shiny beak, no powder on your hands).
- Abnormal feather growth.
- Loss of primary flights and tail.
- Twisted, deformed feathers.

PBFD can also appear in very young nestlings, although it is usually seen in older birds as they begin to wean, or at their first major moult.

In the early stages of the disease, infection underruns their beak. They often will scream to be fed but be unable to chew properly. At this stage the beak may appear normal. As time progresses the beak will become deformed and very long. The underside of the upper beak will become rotten.

This is a slow, cruel disease. The onset of signs is not sudden but they slowly show signs of illness and deteriorate. These birds may have deformed or missing feathers. Closely inspect the powder down feathers near the hip – they should be fluffy and cover the skin. If they are present as tiny 'sticks' and the skin is easy to see, be suspicious of PBFD.

The loss of the powder down feathers means there is no powder in the plumage so they look 'dirty'. As well, they may have shiny beaks – in normal birds the powder makes the beak look dull.

These birds commonly develop signs of secondary infections such as diarrhoea or respiratory disease, as their immune system is depressed. They cannot function to fight disease as well as a normal bird, so diseases that a normal bird could fight off can become a serious threat to their life.

The most commonly affected parrots are cockatoos (eg Sulphur-crested, Corellas, Galahs) and African Grey Parrots, although, any parrot species may be affected.

Papillomatosis
Signs:
Warty growth seen on:
- Feet.
- Preen gland.
- Corner and inside of mouth.
- Around beak.
- Wing.
- Eyelids.
- Cloaca.
- Intestines.

This problem is thought to be caused by a virus but this has not yet been definitely proven. It is very uncommon in Australia despite being very common overseas, particularly in the USA.

The form occurring in the mouth is more common in Green-winged Macaws and Scarlet Macaws. In these birds, the growths can block the opening of the windpipe. In Amazon Parrots it is more common to see the papillomas in the cloaca and will be seen when they hang out during a cloacal prolapse.

Treatment is either surgical removal or application of human wart preparations if the position is such that it can be applied without causing damage to the surrounding structures. Many birds appear to recover if left alone or after treatment and surgery. This can be misleading as some of these birds will develop other tumours internally, especially around the liver and bile duct, or will have recurring tumours in the cloaca. Only two cases have been reported in Australia.

Poxvirus

This virus is more of a problem in young birds, however, it can occasionally be found in older birds. Some reports state that the virus can live on the ground and surrounding areas for up to two years.

Poxvirus causes some different symptoms based on where the virus attacks. The form affecting the skin is commonly called 'Dry Pox'. The form affecting the mouth, throat and windpipe is called 'Wet Pox'. There is also an uncommon form where the virus enters the bloodstream and causes a septicaemia. The different forms can occur in an outbreak in a collection at the same time.

Birds that recover from Poxvirus will normally have protection lasting up to eight months. Vaccination is available in Australia for pigeons only, but there is a parrot poxvirus vaccine available for birds overseas. Vaccines should only be used on healthy flocks – if it is used in the face of an outbreak it may make the disease more severe.

Dry Pox
Signs:
* Red oozing sores around unfeathered areas of skin.

As the disease progresses the sores become large and scabby, then drop off without leaving large scars. Bacteria and fungi will often cause secondary infections.

This is common in raptors, waterfowl, pigeons and passerines (eg Currawong, Magpie, Magpie Lark, canary) but not parrots.

The virus cannot penetrate intact skin so it relies on damage from scratches or mosquito bites to allow it to enter.

Wet Pox
Signs:
* Grey to brown accumulations of cheesy pus in the mouth, throat or windpipe.

If the cheesy pus is removed, there is usually significant bleeding. The birds cannot swallow food well and often have problems breathing.

Diseases that have similar signs are: Infection with *Candida* (Thrush); *Trichomonas* (Canker); Aspergillosis; Pigeon Herpesvirus; Amazon Tracheitis virus; as well as Vitamin A deficiency.

This form is common in parrots, quail, pigeons and starlings overseas. It is occasionally seen in Australia. In parrots the most commonly affected birds are Amazon Parrots and macaws.

Septicaemic Pox
Signs:
* Sudden onset of sleepiness, ruffled feathers.
* Heavy breathing.
* Most birds die within three days.

At post-mortem examination the lungs have many pinpoint haemorrhages, there is a build-up of fat in the liver and inflammation of the small intestines. Confirmation of the diagnosis is based on a pathologist examining the tissue samples. This form is rarely seen in birds other than canaries.

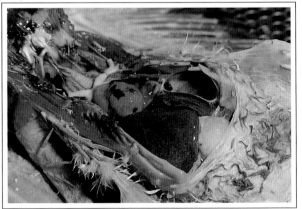

Blood spots (haemorrhages) in heart muscle and other body structures in a juvenile Blue and Gold Macaw with septicaemic pox.

Herpesvirus Infection of the Feet
Signs:
• Warty growths on feet and toes.

There may be warty growths or white patches on the feet of these birds. Once the birds recover there may be permanent loss of pigment in these areas, this being most obvious in birds with dark feet.

Treatment is to use ointments designed to treat cold sores in people. Useful medications are Stoxil™, Herplex™ or Zovirax™.

It is occasionally seen in raptors, cockatoos and macaws.

EXOTIC DISEASES
With the recent outbreak of Newcastle Disease in eastern Australia, mention should be made of two important diseases: Newcastle Disease and Avian Influenza. Both are caused by a virus and have the potential to destroy the poultry industry. If you suspect an exotic disease you can contact AQIS (Australian Quarantine Inspection Service) on freecall 1 800 020 504 or on their Hotline 1 800 803 006

Newcastle Disease Virus
This is a disease of domestic poultry and wild birds. It is caused by a paramyxovirus. The virus can attack the gastrointestinal, respiratory and nervous systems. Depending on the strain of virus, exposure to Newcastle Disease (NDV) may lead to a subclinical infection where the birds show no sign of disease or a range of signs, with mortalities of up to 100%.

Birds of all ages can be infected and mortality rates are highest in young birds.

Natural Hosts
Newcastle Disease can be a highly contagious disease of domestic fowl, ducks, geese, turkeys, guineafowl, quail, pigeons, pheasants and many species of wild and captive birds. All avian species are probably susceptible to Newcastle Disease Virus (NDV), with different species differing in their susceptibilities to a particular NDV strain. Any species can be a source of virus for any other species.

The different bird Orders can be divided into three groups which reflect a general trend in response to NDV:

1. Avian Orders with a **High** Susceptibility to NDV;
   • *Phasianiformes* (gallinaceous birds and pheasants)
   • *Psittaciformes* (parrots)
   • *Struthioniformes* (ratites)
   • *Columbiformes* (pigeons)
2. Avian Orders with an **Intermediate** Susceptibility to NDV;
   • *Strigiformes* (owls)
   • *Falconiformes* (falcons)
   • *Accipitriformes* (eagles)
   • *Ciconiiformes* (storks)
   • *Sphenisciformes* (penguins)
   • *Passeriformes* (sparrows and song birds)
3. Avian Orders with a **Minimal** Susceptibility to NDV;
   • *Anatiformes* (waterfowl)
   • *Pelicaniformes* (pelicans, cormorants)
   • *Ralliformes* (coots and rails)
   • *Lariformes* (gulls)
   • *Carianiformes* (cranes)

As a general rule, birds which have a close association with water are usually resistant to NDV, while granivorous and fructivorous species are moderately susceptible and omnivorous species are most sensitive. Species that gather in flocks are more likely to be affected than solitary species.

Mammals play little or no role in the spread of the virus other than passive transfer. NDV has been shown to cause a mild conjunctivitis in humans.

NDV is not transmitted via eggs as embryos will die before hatching.

In modern poultry sheds, airborne transmission of the virus is accentuated by the use of exhaust fans.

Poultry
The effects will vary with the strength of the virus.

Viscerotropic Velogenic Newcastle Disease (VVND) starts suddenly and progresses rapidly.
Signs:
- Loss of appetite.
- Ruffled feathers.
- Listlessness.
- Blueness and swelling of combs and wattles.
- Watery to pussy eye discharge with conjunctivitis.
- Yellowish green diarrhoea.
- Noisy breathing, sneezing, coughing, nasal discharge and laboured breathing with mouth gaping and extended head and neck.
- Older birds show nervous signs (tremors, neck twisting, incoordination).
- Egg production usually ceases.
- Mortality may reach 100%.

This disease is not present in Australia.

Mesogenic Newcastle Disease is a less severe disease.
Signs:
- Predominantly respiratory and nervous signs present.
- Severe drop in egg production.
- Young are more severely affected.

This disease is not present in Australia.

Lentogenic Newcastle Disease
Signs:
- Mild respiratory problems.
- Egg production drops.
- Negligible to low mortality.

This disease is endemic in Australia

The recent outbreak in eastern Australia was caused by a mutation of one site on the DNA of a Lentogenic form of NDV. This caused the virus to transform into the Velogenic form of NDV. The Lentogenic form had been in Australia for decades without causing any real problem. There is no good explanation as to why it suddenly mutated.

Pigeons:
This disease was first diagnosed in pigeons in the early 1980s and subsequently spread to most parts of the world. Incubation period varies from a few days to five weeks.
Signs:
- Initial sign is increased water intake and urination, watery to bloody diarrhoea followed by nervous signs (head tremor, twisted neck, paralysis of wings and/or legs, poor vision (bird pecks at but misses food).
- Poor feathering if during a moult.
- Respiratory signs always absent.

- Affects 30 –100% of the flock, mortality rate is usually low.
- Convalescence for up to 6 months and may have persistent diarrhoea.

All viruses isolated were PMV-1 serotype.

This disease can transmit to poultry.

Gamebirds and Turkeys:

Pheasants, quail and partridges are more susceptible than guineafowl and turkeys. Usually an outbreak in these birds follows an outbreak in chickens.

Wild Waterfowl:

These birds will usually be exposed to NDV during their annual migration. They do not develop clinical signs but remain carriers for long periods. It is suspected that transmission occurs when they gather in large numbers prior to or during migration.

Velogenic viruses have not been isolated from wild aquatic birds. A form of the virus, that causes no signs in the birds, has been isolated from waterfowl and pelagic seabirds in Western Australia.

Domestic Pet Birds:

Signs are the same as in poultry. The outcome will vary with virulence, dosage and method of entry, age, levels of resistance, presence of passive or active antibodies and levels of stress or concurrent disease.

Outbreaks attributed to pet birds were associated with movement from an infected area during an outbreak – often with smuggled birds. It has often been assisted by the rapid movement of birds due to international air transport, allowing birds to be moved while incubating NDV.

It is not known how these birds become infected with VVND but it is thought to accompany the stress and hygiene breakdown associated with transport. Psittacines can carry and excrete virus for up to 430 days.

Diagnosis

This disease may be suspected but it is impossible to diagnose unequivocally on clinical signs and pathology as it is similar to so many other diseases, such as:
- Virulent Avian Influenza
- Mareks Disease
- Encephalomalacia
- Thiamine deficiency
- Avian Cholera
- Avian Encephalomyelitis

Treatment

This is not permitted in Australia. Any outbreak must be reported to the Federal Department of Agriculture who would handle slaughter and disposal of flocks as well as disinfection of premises and local environment and quarantine procedures. The federal government has a specific plan, called AUSVETPLAN, administered with the co-operation of all states to handle this.

Avian Influenza Virus Type A

Avian Influenza (AI) has been associated with a lethal disease in poultry since 1901. It was first identified as a specific influenza virus in 1955. There have been reported outbreaks of AI in Victoria and Queensland over the past decade.

There are several types of influenza virus. All AI viruses belong to the type A influenza group. The B and C groups affect only humans.

All the subtypes of influenza A virus have been isolated from waterfowl, where it causes minimal intestinal infections. Despite showing no clinical signs, these birds excrete the virus from their respiratory tract, tears and in their droppings. The incubation period can be as short as a few hours and can affect birds of all ages. There is no problem with transmission via eggs as the embryos die prior to hatching.

Influenza viruses differ from other animal viruses in that the RNA is replicated and included in the virus as eight separate single-strand segments. This segmentation of the RNA allows genetic recombination to occur during mixed infection with different influenza A strains, yielding a potential 256 genetically different types of virus. This explains why there are so many different types of virus identified and they all have different effects on the patients as some viruses are stronger than others. Genetic reassortment between human and avian viruses has been suggested as the mechanism by which new human epidemic strains of influenza arise.

Natural Hosts

This is a highly contagious disease of domestic fowl, ducks, geese, turkeys, guineafowl, quail and pheasants. It may be carried by wild birds, particularly waterfowl and seabirds but they usually exhibit no signs.

Signs:

The virus affects all tissues, including the heart. The resulting decrease in heart function results in fluid swelling throughout the body, most evident under the skin.

The signs will vary with factors such as species of bird, age, sex, concurrent diseases, environmental factors and the virulence of the virus.

Acute high virulence virus:
- Sudden death.
- No visible signs or lesions.
- Mortality can be 100% of the flock.

Less virulent virus:
- Ruffled feathers.
- Depression. The bird sits or stands in a semi-comatose state with head touching the ground.
- Loss of appetite.
- Decreased egg production, initially laying soft-shelled eggs and then stopping laying.
- Mild to severe coughing and sneezing.
- Breathing may be laboured.
- Increased tears.
- Swelling and blue colouration of the head, comb and wattles – may have blood spots at the tip of the comb or wattles.
- Haemorrhage may be present in unfeathered areas of the skin.
- Profuse, watery diarrhoea and increased thirst.
- Nervous signs usually occur only in adults.

Diagnosis

This virus may be suspected but it is impossible to diagnose unequivocally on clinical signs and pathology as it is similar to so many other diseases, such as:
- Newcastle Disease
- Mycoplasmosis
- Fowl Cholera
- Chlamydiosis

Treatment

This is not permitted in Australia. Any outbreak must be reported to the Department of Agriculture who will handle slaughter and disposal of flocks as well as disinfection of premises and local environment and quarantine procedures. Refer to AUSVETPLAN for guidelines at www.aabc.com.au/ausvetplan or phone 02 6232 5522 or AQIS on freecall 1 800 803 006.

Control
- Use of vaccines are prohibited in Australia.
- Prevent access of wild birds to poultry sheds, feed stores and water supply.
- Use accepted principles of biosecurity and good management.

Biosecurity Measures
- Only essential workers and vehicles should enter the farm area.
- Provide clean clothing and disinfection facilities for employees.
- Clean and disinfect vehicles (including tyres) entering and leaving the farm.
- Avoid visiting other poultry farms.
- Do not exchange equipment or vehicles with other farms.
- Maintain an 'all-in/all-out' philosophy of farm management.
- Control the movement of all poultry and poultry products from farm to farm.
- Never 'skim' mature birds from a flock for sale to a live poultry market.
- Thoroughly clean and disinfect poultry houses between each lot of birds.
- Prevent contact with wild or migratory birds.
- Do not use water that may have been contaminated by wild birds.

Birds taken to Markets:
- Use plastic rather than wooden crates to aid cleaning.
- Keep scales and floor clean of manure, feathers and other debris.
- Disinfect all equipment, crates and vehicles **before** returning them to the farm.
- Keep incoming poultry separate from unsold birds.
- Clean and disinfect the marketplace after every day of sale.

These measures can be used in combating all the exotic diseases.

NON-INFECTIOUS DISEASES

Feather Picking
Signs:
- Excessive chewing of feathers or skin.
- Normal feathers on head and neck.
- Damaged feathers on easily reached sections of the body.

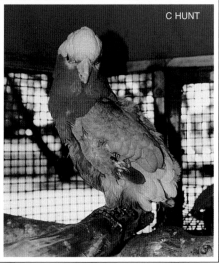
Feather plucked Galah.

This is a common problem in pet birds that are strongly bonded to a person. It is obsessive behaviour and is a sign that the bird is upset – similar to people who chew their fingernails when stressed. It can be seen in any spoilt, handraised bird that has not been properly socialised.

Confusion in diagnosis arises because the same signs can be seen in birds with other disorders such as boredom, fear, breeding frustration, liver diseases, poisoning, malnutrition, infections (bacteria, virus, fungi) and allergies. Some birds will have damaged feathers caused by their mate. There will usually be damaged feathers around the head and neck. This is common in cockatoos.

As the problem progresses the bird will move its attention from the feathers and damage the skin. This is seen as bleeding and areas of ulceration. It can be a difficult problem to identify the cause of the feather picking. Often blood tests are required to determine any infections or internal diseases.

Treatment is a problem as the picking becomes a well-entrenched habit. The list of suggested treatments is very long. Obviously, any infection needs to be treated with antibiotics. Using bitter agents to stop the birds chewing is not very successful. It does not treat the real cause, so the underlying problem is still present.

If the problem has a psychological cause, you need a good imagination and dedication to find ways to help the bird settle down and recover. Tape recordings or the radio, finding someone to 'bird-sit', providing new toys or challenges, moving the bird to a new location are all ideas that you can try. It is difficult to predict the outcome of anything you try. Something that will help one bird settle will make another bird more stressed and increase the feather picking. Hormones and anti-anxiety drugs have been tried with success in some cases.

As a last resort, especially if the bird is causing damage to its skin, is to use an Elizabethan Collar or neck brace.

The species most prone to feather picking are African Grey Parrots, conures, cockatoos (especially Gang Gangs, Galahs and Sulphur-crested Cockatoos) and macaws.

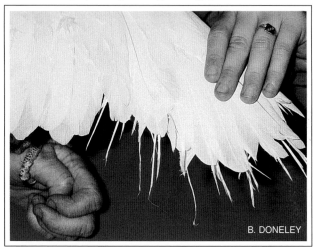

Mutilated wings of a Sulphur-crested Cockatoo feather plucker.

Mutilation Syndrome

Signs:
- Ulcers/bleeding on the wing web and legs.
- Bird constantly chewing at wing web and legs.

There are many theories as to the cause of this problem. It is similar to the Psittacine Pruritic Polyfolliculosis described previously. Many people suspect a virus is the cause. In some cases a Poxvirus or a Herpesvirus has been suggested. It is thought that the chewing is a response to the tingling feeling that some viruses cause (eg Herpesvirus/cold sores in humans).

Treatment is using Elizabethan Collars or neck braces as well as antibiotics. Many will recover with this treatment, but break down again in three to four months.

This is commonly seen overseas in Yellow-naped Amazons, Double Yellow-headed Amazons, Severe Macaws and Yellow-collared Macaws.

Chronic Egg Laying and Egg Binding

Signs:
- Erect posture (penguin-like).
- Straining to lay egg.
- Swollen abdomen.
- Can feel the egg near the vent. Soft-shelled eggs are difficult to feel.

It is common that some birds will lay a large number of eggs. Some of the hens appear to be egg

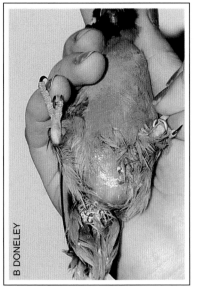

An egg-bound lovebird.

factories, particularly if they have no mate. Egg binding can be a common result of such prolific egg laying as eventually the hen will deplete her reserves of energy and calcium. Do not keep removing the eggs as they are laid or she will continue to lay more. A simple trick is to remove the eggs and hard-boil them and replace them. This will allow them to last while she settles down to her nesting and breaks the cycle. Changing the light pattern by several hours, will often break the cycle as well.

The causes of egg binding include obesity, a diet deficient in calcium, chilling, lack of exercise and infection in the oviduct.

Many birds will respond to being placed in a warm, humid environment and being given a calcium supplement, such as 0.1ml per 100 gram body weight of Calcium Sandoz Syrup™ every 1–2 hours, until the egg is passed. If the hen is weak or depressed she will need veterinary treatment that will range from sucking out the egg contents with a needle and syringe and collapsing the egg, through to surgery similar to a caesarean. As well, the veterinarian will provide fluid therapy and other medications to control infection and to aid the passage of the egg.

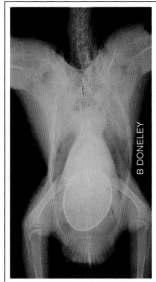

X-Ray of parrot showing egg binding.

In some birds the egg is not in the oviduct but has been laid internally. In these cases, the bird will look similar to an egg-bound bird but you will be unable to feel the egg near the vent. Often the abdomen will be quite swollen and full of fluid. One of the major problems with these birds is that the yolk that is laid internally is prone to developing infection and peritonitis will develop. This is life threatening and needs prompt veterinary treatment if the bird is to survive.

Yolk Stroke
Signs:
- Convulsions.
- Paralysis.
- Sitting on the floor and not moving.
- Head twisted to the side or backwards.

This may follow a yolk that has been laid internally. The fat, from the yolk, is absorbed from the abdominal cavity into the blood vessels. The clot of fat is washed away and blocks a blood vessel supplying the brain. The bird will appear to have suffered a stroke. Take the bird to your veterinarian immediately.

Yolk Peritonitis
Signs:
- Slow onset of lethargy.
- Swelling of the abdomen.
- Hen has laid eggs recently or is due to lay eggs.
- Tail bobbing.

This is commonly seen in Cockatiels, African Lovebirds, Budgerigars, waterfowl, doves and occasionally in Scarlet Macaws (it is rare in Blue and Gold Macaws and Green-winged Macaws). However, it can occur in any egg-laying hen if the yolk misses the oviduct and spills into the abdomen. This is a potentially lethal disease. In some birds the first sign seen is sudden death.

The most common diagnostic procedure is to collect the fluid from the abdomen into a syringe. In egg yolk peritonitis, the fluid is often golden in colour, just like a yolk. This is then examined with a microscope.

Blood tests can help assess the level of damage that has occurred inside the bird's abdomen. In some cases, the bird (especially Cockatiels) will become a diabetic because of damage to its pancreas. This is usually temporary. A small number of birds may have signs of a 'stroke' from egg yolk absorbed into the bloodstream.

Treatment is normally what is required for a critical bird – fluid therapy, warmth and humidity, antibiotics and anti-inflammatory injections. Some birds may need surgery to remove the excessive fluid and flush out the abdomen.

Long-term treatment, in birds with this as a recurring problem, is removal of the oviduct – similar to desexing a dog or cat. Because this is such a prevalent problem in pet Cockatiels, some avian veterinarians routinely recommend desexing them at a young age (6–12 months). Once they are desexed, the birds will no longer lay eggs. The ovary does not fully develop the yolks but some of the hens will show signs of abdominal cramps during the normal breeding season.

Congenital Eye Deformity

Signs:
• Incomplete separation of eyelids.
• Narrow eyelids.

This is usually an inherited problem, so the parents should be separated and the mating not repeated. Use records of subsequent matings with other birds to decide who to cull from your breeding program. It is more commonly seen in the Lutino variety but can occur in any colour. Surgery has been performed on many of these birds but is not usually successful. With time they learn to cope very well and can make excellent pets. These birds should definitely not be used for breeding.

Cockatiel Conjunctivitis

Signs:
• Watery eye discharge.
• Swollen, inflamed conjunctiva.
• Swollen eyelids.
• Partial eyelid paralysis.
• Weak jaw tone.

This is a problem seen more commonly in Lutino varieties of Cockatiels. It appears to be more common in some family lines and is regarded as being an inherited problem. Despite many tests no infectious cause has been identified. One theory is that it is a response to glare because these birds lack pigment in their iris and retina.

Treatment is to avoid glare by keeping the Lutino birds in shady aviaries. Eye ointments can be applied very sparingly to reduce the inflammation. Discuss this with your veterinarian. Recurrence of the problem is common.

Macaw 'Acne'

Signs:
• Small swellings on the face.

This is caused by small, ingrown feathers on the face and eyelids of macaws.

These birds often need simple surgery to release the trapped feathers as well as antibiotic injections. In some cases, injections of corticosteroids are needed if the birds are rubbing or scratching at the affected sites.

The problem is most commonly seen in Blue and Gold Macaws, Scarlet Macaws and Green-winged Macaws.

Injuries

Signs:
• Fractures to legs or wings.
• Bruising.

- Cuts.
- Feather loss or damage.

This is more common in pet birds that are allowed free flight in the home. It may also result from panic. Birds are easily injured by cats, doors, stoves, hot water, toilets, slammed doors etc. Treatment depends upon the area and extent of damage. The main point of concern is that this problem should be preventable. You must take steps to avoid situations where the bird will be exposed to circumstances where it can be injured.

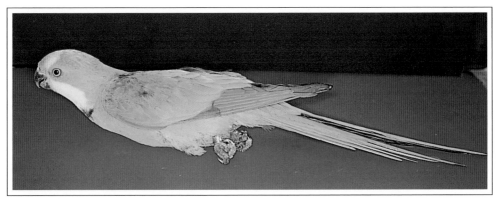

Polyteline Paralysis in a Superb Parrot cock. This a form of paralysis seen in parrots, but particularly in the Polytelis genus.

Paralysis Syndrome
Signs:
- Trembling.
- Wobbly gait.
- Incoordination.
- Reluctant to walk.
- Lying on the floor of the cage.
- Abnormal head movements.

This syndrome in Cockatiels has been reported in the USA but has not been seen in Australia. It is thought to be associated with a Vitamin E and selenium deficiency. This form of malnutrition is related to intestinal damage caused by *Giardia* infection.

If the patient is in the early stages of the disease, treatment with injectable selenium and injectable or oral Vitamin E supplement may be successful. Once the disease is advanced, treatment is unlikely to be successful.

There is a syndrome seen in parrots, particularly the members of the *Polytelis* genus: Superb Parrot *Polytelis swainsonii*, Regent Parrot *P. anthopeplus* and Princess Parrot *P. alexandrae*. The birds have clenching of both feet, their legs are drawn under their body and they cannot stand up. In some cases the wings are affected as well. There is no successful medication for these birds other than using physiotherapy by bicycling the legs and clenching and unclenching the feet. This should be done several times daily. The sooner the physiotherapy is begun the more likely the birds will recover. Place the bird on soft bedding which should be changed when it becomes soiled. Provide food and water containing electrolytes. A virus has been suspected as causing this syndrome but none has been identified.

Lutino Cockatiel Syndrome
Signs:
- Baldness (especially on the crown of head).
- Haemophiliac (prone to uncontrolled bleeding).
- More prone to disease.

- Appear to be mentally retarded/undeveloped.
- Incoordination (appear drunk).
- Fall off the perch at night.
- Bruising and bleeding of the wing tip, wrist, abdomen and pectoral muscles from trauma/falling over.

In the USA there are a lot of genetic problems with Lutino Cockatiels. So much so, that they have been given a special name to the mixture of signs that can be seen. Some or all of the signs above may be present. While we do have some of the problems in Australia, they do not occur very frequently.

Since the cause of these problems is inherited, there is no treatment. Night lights may avoid the panic that occurs in these birds when they fall off their perch at night.

Euthanasia should be performed on severely affected birds.

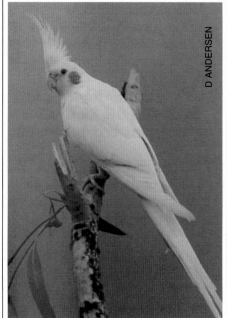

Lutino Cockatiel.

Wing Tumours
Signs:
- Swelling or a mass appearing anywhere on the wing.
- Tumours may develop and be seen as large masses in muscles or skin on the wings.

These can be tumours arising from the muscle or from the bone. The only treatment is surgery and this is often amputation. It is best performed as soon as the lump is detected.

Gout
Signs:
- Depression.
- Lameness in one or both feet.
- Swelling of joints (redness and white substance present in joints).

The major waste product contained in the urates is nitrogen. This is why the urates appear as a white paste in the droppings. When the kidneys don't function well this nitrogen (urates) builds up in the blood. To remove the build-up, the urates are deposited into any area the body can find. Usually this is into joints or around the heart, liver and internal organs. This condition is called gout. When it occurs in joints, it is called articular gout and when it occurs inside the body it is called visceral gout. Why it occurs in one site in some birds and another site in other birds is not known.

The most common cause of gout is old age or advanced kidney disease, but it can also be seen with severe dehydration – a good reason to ensure your birds always have plenty of fresh water available.

This disease can be confirmed during a visit to your avian veterinarian, who will examine the bird's urine or use blood tests to

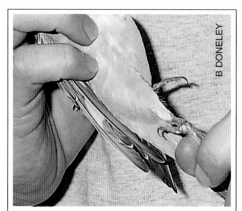

Gout in Budgerigar.

confirm the kidney problems underlying the gout.

All birds with kidney disease need fluid therapy (see *Fluid Therapy – Electrolytes* on page 20). As well, allopurinol (Zyloprim™), a drug which helps dissolve the urates and aid in their excretion, is used. The long term outlook for these birds is poor. Euthanasia should be considered if they are very ill.

Feather Cysts
Signs:
- Swellings on the body wall, wings or tail.

This is due to an abnormal feather growing underneath the skin instead of coming out of the feather follicle as normal. It may be an inherited problem in many birds, but other causes have been suggested including injury to feather follicle, malnutrition, parasites, viral or bacterial infections.

The usual treatment is surgery to remove the damaged follicle. If the feather is simply cut and removed, it will usually return with the same problem at a later date.

This is most commonly seen in Blue and Gold Macaws and Norwich and Gloster Canaries.

Liver Failure
Signs:
- Weakness.
- Wobbly gait (as if drunk).
- Difficulty breathing.
- Swollen abdomen (full of fluid).
- Swollen liver.

The liver is an extremely important organ and can be affected by many diseases. The problem occurs because the bird may not show any signs until nearly all the liver has been damaged. This is referred to as an 'end-stage' liver.

Causes can be cancer, fat infiltration from a high fat diet or cirrhosis from chronic exposure to a wide variety of poisons. X-rays and blood tests will help to identify the cause and give an indication of how severe the problem may be.

Treatment is usually euthanasia as the bird's condition is often untreatable by the time it begins to show signs.

Dislocated Knee
Signs:
- Seen in young birds prior to fledging.
- Legs appear twisted and deformed from the knee down.

It is suspected that this is a congenital birth defect. As the bird develops, it becomes obvious that it has a deformity in one or both legs. On close inspection you will see that there is a twisting of the leg below the knee.

Treatment has been attempted using splints, bandages and surgery but is usually unsuccessful.

This condition would make you consider culling the parents from your breeding program.

Red Mite
Signs:
- Skin irritation.
- Pale legs or beak (anaemia).
- Excessive scratching.
- Poor feather condition.

This mite is not specific to any particular group of birds but will feed on any bird it finds. Usually they occur in large numbers. They hide in cracks in the walls, and other parts of the environment, during the day. At night they come out and suck blood from the bird. In some cases, they remove so much blood from the bird that anaemia occurs. Eventually this can lead to death – especially in nestlings.

Treatment is lightly dusting the birds and nesting material with Carbaryl™ or pyrethrin powder. As well the aviary or cage can be sprayed with a mixture of a soluble pyrethrin (eg Coopex™) to saturate and penetrate into all the small cracks that protect the mites during the day.

These mites are a common problem in canaries and other passerines.

Abnormal Behaviour

This problem is more common in pet birds. Each bird has its own personality. As they grow and develop this becomes more evident particularly in pet birds that have been handreared. Many of the birds we keep as pets have an instinct to be with a mate or as part of a flock. When pet birds become bonded to you, they expect you to fill this role. They want you to be present all the time. If their needs are not met, they can often develop habits that are annoying.

Screaming

Pet conures, macaws and large cockatoos develop the habit of screaming when they are upset. This is not a phase they are going through, but it will progressively get worse until it is unbearable. Some birds will screech and scream for hours at a time.

To treat this you need to identify the times of day that it usually occurs. Begin a training or play session just prior to this time. If this is not possible, place the bird in a different, dark location just prior to this time. Resist the temptation of screaming at the bird to 'be quiet' from another room. This teaches the bird that it is a good thing for you to scream at each other and reinforces that screaming is acceptable. Birds learn that screaming is a wonderful way to attract their owner's attention. You need to train yourself not to react as this also reinforces the behaviour. It may not be possible to totally eliminate screaming but you can encourage the bird to replace it with less noisy alternatives.

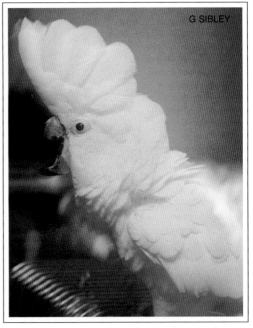

A Moluccan Cockatoo letting loose.

Spend some time observing the bird to see if something in particular triggers the screaming. Does he always scream at a particular time of day or in a special location? You need to discover when, where and why your bird is screaming. This will allow you to anticipate the screaming episodes. Once identified you can either remove the trigger or offer a distraction just before the trigger occurs. If the bird screams just before you leave the room, you can provide a food treat or ring his bell loudly so that he will mimic this as you leave, ie he will distract himself with his bell rather than scream. You need to train the bird to reward itself by concentrating on a distraction when it does not scream. If the bird learns that not screaming will bring a reward, it is motivated to avoid screaming. Other distractions include providing a bath; giving exercise (flying or a chasing game) so that he is not suffering an overabundance of energy; spraying a water mist above the bird (not directly at the bird) so that it settles onto the bird as a fine mist, like rain – this will often distract the bird and encourage a calm state that is usually followed by grooming to remove the excess water; changing the feeding time to occur just before a trigger time; introducing a new toy. This is a hard and time-consuming problem to correct.

Social Regurgitation
To show it really cares about you, the bird will regurgitate food to you. This may be mistaken as vomiting and illness. In reality, it is a sign of deep affection and is what bonded pairs of birds do for each other. It can be a common sign in macaws, Budgerigars and cockatoos.

Severe Aggression during Breeding Season
Many birds that have become strongly bonded to people become very possessive. Some birds become aggressive towards anyone who approaches their 'mate' during the breeding season. They may fly and attack the head and face of a 'rival'. The problem needs to be overcome in the early stages as once it is well-established it is very difficult to remove.

Nutritional Problems
High-fat Content in Diet
Signs:
- Overweight.
- Lethargic.
- Weak.
- Liver lipidosis. Fat damages the liver and causes sudden death from liver failure.

This is common in birds on a high-fat seed diet, eg sunflower and safflower. You need to wean these birds onto a healthier diet. Change their diet to Budgerigar seed mix or wean the bird onto one of the high quality parrot pellets which are more balanced and include fruit and vegetables.

Calcium Deficiency
In young birds
- Fractures occur in bones from normal day-to-day events.
- Soft bones.
- Beak easily bent.
In adult birds
- Poor egg production.
- Egg binding.

The levels of calcium in the bird's blood are controlled by the parathyroid gland, a tiny gland in the neck. Problems with this gland can cause variations in the blood calcium level. Provide a calcium supplement and improve the bird's diet.

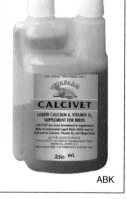

ABK

Calcivet™ – a liquid calcium supplement.

Hypocalcaemia
Signs:
- Weakness.
- Falling from perch.
- Poor gripping of perch.
- Convulsions.
- Uncontrolled flapping of wings.

African Grey Parrots have lower blood levels of calcium than other parrots. The level of calcium in a bird's blood is controlled by the parathyroid gland. Calcium is an important chemical for the normal functioning of the nervous system. If the blood levels of calcium drop too low, the birds will show signs that the nervous system is not functioning normally. In the early stages the birds look uncoordinated and clumsy. As time progresses they become weak and have trouble gripping their perch well. They often fall from the perch – particularly if excited or suddenly frightened.

The level of calcium in the blood can be measured by a simple laboratory test.

The exact cause of this problem in African Grey Parrots is still uncertain. Many of these birds have been on a diet deficient in calcium and Vitamin D3. Usually this is an all-seed diet. In some cases, it is thought that a virus has infected the parathyroid gland as the parathyroid glands are often enlarged at post-mortem examination.

Prevention is best achieved by removing high-fat seeds from the diet and replacing them with calcium supplements and dairy products. High-fat seeds actually interfere with the absorption of calcium from the intestine.

Adequate levels of Vitamin A should also be provided. This can be done with a vitamin supplement in the drinking water or by providing plenty of green, leafy vegetables.

It is important that the levels of calcium in the diet are in balance with the phosphorus content. The recommended calcium to phosphorus ratio for birds is 2:1. All seeds are low in calcium so a diet that is made up mostly of seeds causes a calcium deficiency. Foods containing high levels of calcium are bones, cheese and yoghurt – you can use these or as an alternative, add calcium to the diet by using powders or syrups. Many birds will improve if weaned onto parrot pellets.

Metabolic Bone Disease
Signs:
• Spontaneous fractures/bending of legs and wings.

This is usually a problem in young birds during their growing stage. They need balanced levels of calcium and phosphorus in their food. They also need adequate levels of Vitamin D3 which helps the absorption of calcium by the intestines.

Birds fed a diet of only seeds, or some handrearing mixes, will not receive enough calcium. In the same way, birds raised indoors without exposure to sunlight will not form enough Vitamin D3. In both these situations, the birds will develop soft bones. As the bones become softer, they are not strong enough to support the normal wear and tear. Eventually these bones will bend and become deformed. The first fractures usually occur in the legs. These are painful and the birds sit awkwardly. To move around they then use their wings. This puts a lot of weight onto the wing bones and they then will bend and deform.

Hens may also show this problem when they are egg laying, as the eggshell takes a lot of calcium from the bird. These birds become weak, lay soft-shelled eggs and may have convulsions.

To help with this problem you need to closely examine the diet. In advanced cases, calcium injections may be required. In the early stages, you need to balance the calcium and phosphorus in the diet. Many foods are low in calcium and high in phosphorus.

Food	Calcium	:	Phosphorus
Millet	1.0	:	6
Peanuts	1.0	:	6
Sunflower	1.0	:	7
Oats	1.0	:	8
Milo	1.0	:	14
Corn	1.0	:	37
Yoghurt	1.6	:	1
Cheese	1.2	:	1
Meat	1.0	:	20

To overcome Vitamin D3 deficiency, you need to give the bird exposure to sunlight each day. As well, you can buy vitamin supplements to add to food or water. Check the label carefully that it contains Vitamin D3 and not other forms of Vitamin D. Birds must receive the D3 form of Vitamin D.

Be careful you do not give too much Vitamin D3 or calcium, as an excess can cause as many problems as a deficiency. If you are not sure, take a list of the ingredients you wish to use in a diet and let your avian veterinarian help you work out a balanced formulation.

Vitamin A Deficiency

Signs:

- Prone to respiratory infections.
- Swellings and abscesses in the mouth and around the tongue.
- Stress prone.
- Die with handling.

If a bird is fed an all-seed diet, it will suffer from malnutrition as this diet is low in Vitamin A and calcium and high in fat.

It has been common in the past to feed high-fat seeds as a major component of the diet (eg sunflower, saf-flower and peanuts).

Examination and correction of any faults in the diet is the best treatment. Offer and encourage your bird to eat a varied diet that contains a wide range of greens, fruit and vegetables as well as parrot pellets. If they are not keen to eat, just provide seed for 10 to 15 minutes twice a day, then at other times provide a wide range of fruit, greens and vegetables in the same dish as the one seed is normally placed in. This lets them know that this is food.

Suitable fruit, greens and vegetables should

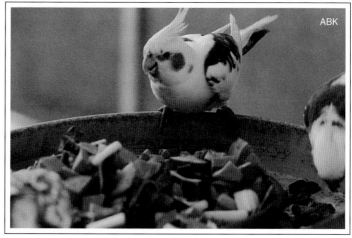

Above: Offer and encourage your bird to eat a varied diet that contains a wide range of greens, fruit and vegetables. Below: Purple-crowned Fruit Dove offered a varied diet.

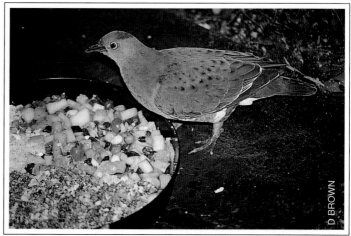

include apple, endive, tomato, peach, celery, cotoneaster, pear, carrot, raisins, plum, corn, sultanas, grape, peas, currants, mango, beans, loquat, paw-paw, silverbeet, nectarine, orange, spinach, figs, strawberry, sprouted mung beans, raspberries, kiwi fruit, native grasses, apricots, rockmelon, parsley, honeydew melon.

While this is not an exhaustive list, it gives you a lot to choose from and to select other similar foods. Provide only a small amount of broccoli. Avoid avocado, rhubarb, cabbage, brussel sprouts and cauliflower. Lettuce is a waste of time for any bird unless it is on a weight-loss diet as it really only contains water and fibre, which is of very little nutritional value.

Flowers from Australian native trees and shrubs such as *Grevillea*, *Acacia* (wattle) and *Callistemon* (bottlebrush) are also appreciated. Some birds enjoy rose petals which are quite safe, however, as a general rule avoid branches or flowers from non-native plants. These include many of the popular indoor plants.

Animal protein can be supplied to the bird as eggs, boiled or scrambled, small pieces of meat or a plain cake such as madeira cake. Also, wholegrain or wholemeal bread can be used as a supplement. Provide a calcium supplement to handreared birds and to hens during the courtship period prior to nesting. Vitamin A injections should be a consideration for any bird with respiratory problems if they are on a poor diet.

Suitable parrot pellets include Vetafarm™, Pretty Bird™, Roudybush™, Harrison's™ and Passwell's™.

Diabetes Mellitus
Signs:
- Excessive thirst and eating.
- Depression.
- Weakness.
- Excess urine.
- Swollen abdomen.

This is a case of 'sugar' diabetes and is the same as in humans. In birds it is only occasionally a problem. It may be seen with egg peritonitis where the pancreas has been damaged. In these cases it is usually only a temporary problem and treatment is usually not required. Your veterinarian will be able to diagnose this by running tests on samples of urine and blood.

Goitre
Signs:
- Vomiting.
- Heavy breathing (tail bobbing).
- Noisy breathing (cheeping).
- Dry retching or neck stretching.

This is a common problem in Budgerigars fed a diet deficient in iodine. The iodine deficiency causes the thyroid gland to enlarge up to five times its normal size. This places pressure on the oesophagus and windpipe. These birds cannot empty their crop effectively and have trouble breathing.

To prevent this problem, you can add iodine to the drinking water. Use one drop of Lugol's Iodine™ in 30ml of water. This should be available to the bird once a week. The Lugol's Iodine™, (or a close relative, Gram's Iodine™), is available from most chemists or your avian veterinarian. An alternative is to place a clump of grass and dirt on the floor. Most soils contain iodine and this is the natural way a Budgerigar finds its iodine requirement.

In advanced cases the bird needs thyroid hormone, as well as iodine, in its drinking water.

Problems Associated with Chewing
All birds love to chew, particularly those allowed to fly around the home. This may cause a problem if they chew the wrong material.

Heavy Metal Poisoning
Signs:
- Depression.

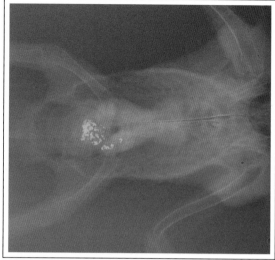

A radiograph of a bird that has chewed the galvanised wire on its aviary. The bright white dots in the abdomen are metal particles. This is the best way to diagnose this problem, which is more common than many people realise.

- Blood in urates or faeces.
- Green or black diarrhoea.
- Vomiting.
- Crop not emptying.
- Convulsions.
- Excessive drinking.
- Excessive urine in droppings.

This type of poisoning is usually from chewing the lead and zinc from galvanised wire. If you have seen your bird chewing this type of wire, mention it to the veterinarian. It may also occur from mercury if the bird chews the back of a mirror. An X-ray or blood tests may be necessary to differentiate this from other poisons. The bird will need hospitalising and treatment with fluid therapy and special injectable medication which removes the heavy metal from the bird's system. With early treatment most birds will survive and recover completely.

Foreign Body Ingestion
Signs:
- Vomiting.
- Enlarged crop.
- Depression.

Because birds like to chew everything and anything, they may take in some material that is too large to pass from the crop. Chewing on fibrous material will cause impaction in the crop where the fibres become entangled and form a mat or ball. This will stop the passage of food and the bird may initially lose weight.

Often the only treatment is surgery to open the crop or stomach and remove the offending material.

Inhaled Seeds/Pus in the Trachea
Signs:
- Wheezing.
- Neck and mouth stretched out.
- Breathing through the mouth.
- Wings held away from the body.
- Severe tail bobbing and movements to breathe.

This is an emergency. It may be caused by a small seed or pus from an infection (bacteria or *Trichomonas*) or by a fungal infection, Aspergillosis. This will

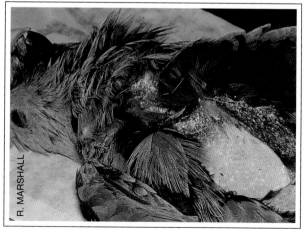

Fungal Aspergillosis obstructing proventriculus in Eclectus.

R. MARSHALL

lodge in the trachea (windpipe) and block the passage of air. If treatment is not given as soon as possible, the bird may die.

The bird will need surgery to dislodge obstruction. To correct its breathing problem a tube is inserted through its side into the abdominal air sacs. Once this tube is in place the bird will immediately settle down and breathe normally. Seeds and pus can be removed under anaesthetic with an endoscope.

If the underlying problem is Aspergillosis, then treatment will be required. It is an extremely difficult disease to treat and the outcome is often unsuccessful. The underlying cause is often stress. If the problem is only the plug in the trachea, treatment may be successful. If there are more problems in the air sacs, then the outlook is poor. Prevention depends upon reducing the number of fungal spores that the birds can inhale. This is best done using bleach on the aviary walls and floor and utensils, especially during the humid months each year.

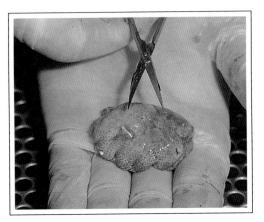

An abscess from inhaled food in the lung of a juvenile Blue and Gold Macaw.

Common Diseases According to Species

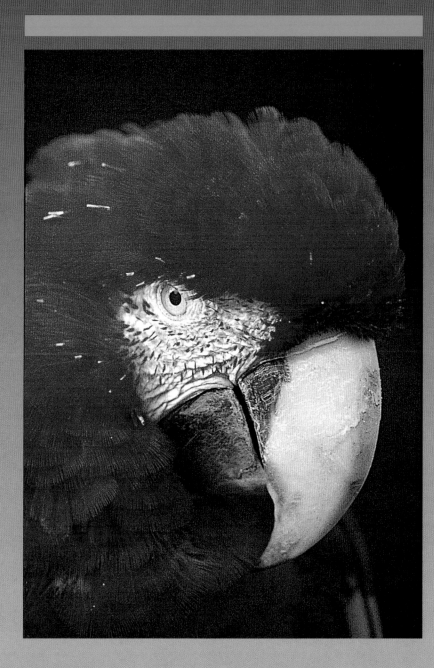

LIST OF COMMON DISEASES
ACCORDING TO SPECIES

Macaws

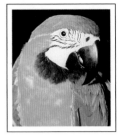

- Abnormal Behaviour.
  - Screaming.
  - Social Regurgitation.
  - Severe Aggression during breeding season.
- Allergic Sinusitis and Bronchitis.
- Feather Cysts (Blue and Gold Macaws).
- Feather Picking.
- Gram Negative Bacterial Infections.
- Hairworm (*Capillaria*).
- Herpesvirus Infection of feet.
- Macaw 'Acne'.
- Mutilation Syndrome (Severe and Yellow-collared Macaws).
- Papillomatosis.
  - Oral and Cloacal (Green-winged and Scarlet Macaws).
- Proventricular Dilatation Disease (PDD).
- Psittacosis.
- Roundworm (*Ascaridia*).
- Sunken Eye Syndrome.
- Toe Constriction Syndrome of young macaws.
- Yolk Peritonitis (Scarlet Macaws).

Asiatic Parrots

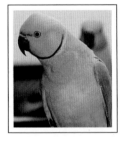

- Aspergillosis.
- Cloacal Prolapse.
- Gram Negative Bacterial Infection.
- Hairworm (*Capillaria*).
- Heavy Metal Poisoning.
- Metabolic Bone Disease in juveniles.
- Megabacteria.
- Nestling Viral Diseases.
- PBFD (*Circovirus*).
- Psittacosis.
- Roundworms (*Ascaridia*).

African Grey Parrots

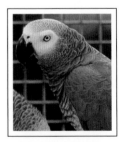

- Abnormal Behaviour.
- Cancer.
- Feather Picking.
- Heavy Metal Poisoning.
- Hypocalcaemia.
- PBFD (*Circovirus*).
- Proventricular Dilatation Disease (PDD).
- Tapeworms.
- Toe Constriction Syndrome.

Conures

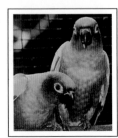

- Conure Bleeding Syndrome.
- Egg binding.
- Feather Picking.
- Gram Negative Bacterial Infection.

- Hairworms (*Capillaria*).
- Pacheco's Disease/Carriers (Patagonian and Nanday Conures).
- Papillomatosis.
- Polyomavirus (Papovavirus).
- Proventricular Dilatation Disease (PDD).
- Psittacosis.

Amazon Parrots

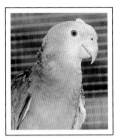

- Abnormal Behaviour.
    - Aggression during mating season.
    - Snuffling.
    - Feather Picking (rare, as they are easily amused).
- Cancer.
- Gram Negative Bacterial Infection.
- Heavy Metal Poisoning.
- Mutilation Syndrome.
- Obesity.
- Papillomatosis.
- Poxvirus.
- Psittacosis.
- Upper Respiratory Disease.
- Vitamin A Deficiency.

Lorikeets/Lories

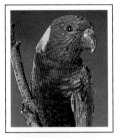

- Fungal Crop Infections.
    - Poor housing, contaminated food.
- Bacterial Septicaemia.
    - Poor housing, contaminated food.
- Nutritional Diseases.
- PBFD (*Circovirus*).
- Paralysis Syndrome.

African Lovebirds

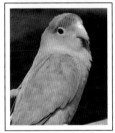

- Bacterial Septicaemia.
- Egg binding.
- Fighting/Trauma from other birds.
- Hairworms (*Capillaria*).
- Megabacteria.
- Roundworms (*Ascaridia*).
- Psittacine Pruritic Polyfolliculosis.
- PBFD (*Circovirus*).
- Psittacosis.
- Upper Respiratory Tract Infections.
- Yolk Peritonitis.

Budgerigars

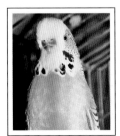

- Trichomoniasis (Canker).
- Scaly-face Mite (*Cnemidocoptes*).
- Coccidiosis.
- Roundworms (*Ascaridia*).
- Hairworms (*Capillaria*).
- French Moult (PBFD/*Circovirus*).
- Bacterial Septicaemias.
- Red Mite in nestboxes.

- Egg binding.
- Cancer (Neoplasia).
- Tumours in kidneys and gonads.
- Goitre.
- Gout (Visceral and Articular).
- Obesity.
- Psittacine Pruritic Polyfolliculosis.

Neophemas
- Conjunctivitis/Psittacosis.
- Roundworms (*Ascaridia*).
- Bacterial Septicaemia.
- Scaly-face Mite (*Cnemidocoptes*), (especially in Scarlet-chested Parrots).

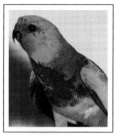

Psephotus
- Roundworms (*Ascaridia*).
- Chilling of nestlings, (especially in Hooded and Golden-shouldered Parrots).
- Injuries – Fighting.
- Conjunctivitus/Psittacosis.

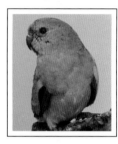

Polytelis
- Roundworms (*Ascaridia*), (especially in Princess Parrots).
- Scaly-face Mite (*Cnemidocoptes*), (especially in Princess Parrots).
- Bacterial Septicaemia.
- Conjunctivitis/Psittacosis. (*Mycoplasma* in Superb Parrots).
- Paralysis Syndrome.

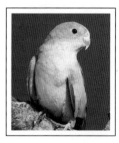

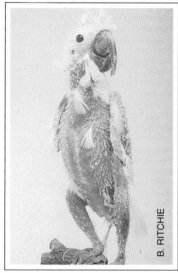

Cockatoos
- Abnormal behaviour.
  - Aggression.
  - Screaming.
  - Feather Picking.
  - Self-mutilation.
- Bacterial Septicaemia.
- Cloacal Prolapse.
- Fungal Crop Infections, (especially black cockatoos).
- Kidney Infections (Nephritis).
- Metabolic Bone Disease in juveniles.
- Obesity.
- PBFD (*Circovirus*).
- Psittacosis.
- Tapeworms.

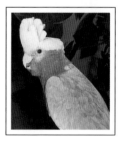

B. RITCHIE

Sulphur-crested Cockatoo with PBFD

Cockatiels

- Bacterial Infection.
- Candidiasis.
- Conjunctivitis/Psittacosis.
- Egg binding.
- *Giardia lamblia.*
- Heavy Metal Poisoning.
- Nutritional Problems.
    - Calcium Deficiency.
    - Obesity.
    - Vitamin A Deficiency.
- Roundworms (*Ascaridia*).
- Upper Respiratory Tract Infections.
- Yolk Stroke.

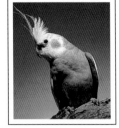

Pigeons

- Upper Respiratory Tract Infections.
- *Trichomonas* (Canker).
- Salmonellosis (*Paratyphoid*).
- Colibacillosis (*E. coli*).
- Chlamydophilosis.
- Roundworm (*Ascaridia*).
- Hairworm or Wireworm (*Capillaria*).
- Lice.
- Red Mite.
- Pigeon Pox.
- Coccidiosis.

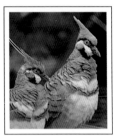

Canaries and Finches

- Air Sac Mite, (especially in the Gouldian Finch and Canary).
- Canary Pox.
- Feather Cysts.
- Egg Peritonitis.
- Coccidiosis.
- Tapeworms.
- Gizzardworms (*Acuaria*).

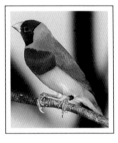

POST-MORTEM EXAMINATION FOR THE AVICULTURIST

Every bird that dies should receive a post-mortem examination or autopsy.
As a bird owner, you are not only interested in the cause of death but are concerned that it may be a contagious disease. You need an answer to help protect the rest of your collection.

You need to approach each examination in an organised manner and must keep good records. The value of the information received from this examination will depend upon the quality of the technique you use. If you are sloppy your results will be confusing and of minimal use. You need to take care and do the examination in a systematic manner so that no lesions are missed. A thorough post-mortem examination will often provide more information than any other diagnostic procedure. If you do not feel capable then take the bird to an experienced avian veterinarian.

I keep a separate set of instruments for post-mortem and have the facilities to carry out most of the simple pathology tests that are relevant. Often the samples collected will be dispatched to an experienced avian veterinary pathologist. This is because many times organs will appear to be normal yet reveal damage and signs of disease when examined under a microscope.

Aims of a Post-mortem Examination

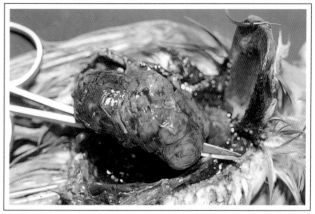

A large tumour occupying most of the abdomen. The bird was having great difficulty breathing as the tumour took up so much space.

To determine:
- The cause of death.
- Progress of the disease.
- Whether the bird had any other problems.
- Whether the worming program was effective.
- Whether feeding and nutrition were adequate.
- Whether the bird was mature and getting ready to breed.

This allows for the examination to be a useful tool to monitor diseases or problems that may affect other birds in a collection. This information monitors the effectiveness of any program to prevent disease. If the program is not effective then changes can be made. Other preventative steps may need to be included. The primary aim should be to use the information gleaned from this post-mortem examination to design management procedures that will remove any problems.

Records

Maintaining a high standard of good records is mandatory. All results of the examination should be written down.

I use a printed form that is half the size of an A4 sheet of paper (so that it can be photocopied on both sides of the sheet and result in two examination forms – see Figure 1. This sheet has all the organs and body systems itemised so that I am less likely to overlook something important. This is filled out by my veterinary nurse as I dictate the results while the examination is being performed. I prefer to use a shorthand system of symbols of arrows up and down to indicate increased or decreased and a subjective system of plus and minus signs to indicate changes in quantity or size. This system can be modified to suit an individual's needs so that +, ++, +++, and ++++ will have relevance to the operator. This is a simple and quick method and overcomes the tendency in a busy practice to put off paperwork because it is time consuming. It is also much easier to quickly scan an examination sheet at a later date.

AVIAN POST-MORTEM EXAMINATION

Name: Street:
Phone: Suburb: Postcode:

Date:. . . . .   Species:. . . . . Age:. . . . . Sex: M F
How long have you had this bird:. . . . . Pet/Aviary; New/Old;
Animal I.D: . . . .   Medications:. . . . .
Diet:. . . . . Recent Deaths: Y N
Species Involved: . . . . History: . . . .

External Features:	Pectoral Muscle	Weight Loss	Dehydration
	Wounds	Skin	Claws
	Eyes	Feathers	Nares
	Fat Deposits	Ears	Soiling
Subcutaneous Tissues:	Peritoneum		
Respiratory System:	Sinuses	Lungs	Trachea
	Upper Airway	Air Sacs	Choana
	Syrinx		
Cardiovascular:	Heart	Blood Vessels	Pericardium
Haematopoietic:	Spleen	Bursa	Thymus
	Bone Marrow		
Digestive System:	Oral Cavity	Beak	Tongue
	Oropharynx	Crop	Oesophagus
	Proventriculus	Gizzard	Small Intestine
	Caecum	Large Intestine	Cloaca
	Liver	Bile Duct	Gall Bladder
	Pancreas	Yolk Sac	
Musculoskeletal:	Muscles	Bones	Joints
Urinary:	Kidney	Ureter	Cloaca

Reproductive:	Gonads	Reproductive tract	
Endocrine:	Pituitary	Thyroid	Parathyroid
	Adrenal Gland		
Nervous:	Brain	Spinal Cord	Periph Nerve

PATHOLOGY (circle)

	Crop Wash	Faecal Float	Intestinal Scrape
	Gram Stain	MZN	Macchiavello/Clearview
Culture:	Heart Blood	Faeces/GIT	

Other (specify)_____ Histopath (specify)_____

	Fee	Credit	Bal

Diagnosis: Definitive Tentative _____

Comments:_____

FIGURE 1

History

All post-mortem examinations begin with as detailed a history as possible. This is extremely important if you do not perform the examination yourself but get your veterinarian to do it. The history helps to explain some of the signs that will be discovered during the examination.

It is vitally important to know:
- Symptoms prior to death.
- Number of ill or dead birds.
- Whether this bird is typical of the current problem.

- Whether the bird was kept with other birds. How many birds and what species?
- Any recent introductions of new birds and their source.
- Whether any medications had been given. If so, what medications and dosage?
- What the normal dietary components were.
- Whether the bird was allowed to roam freely through the house.
- Whether it had been exposed to any toxic substances, eg smoke, cooking fumes, sprays, new paint, indoor plants, ornaments etc.
- Whether the bird had been recently introduced to a new aviary.
- What substrate was used in the aviary/cage.
- Whether predators were a problem on the property.
- Whether any new food, insecticides or disinfectants were used.
- How long had the owner had the bird.
- How long had the bird been dead.
- How had the cadaver been stored since death – frozen or chilled?
- Any other information the owner feels is relevant.

A good history allows you to gather any extra equipment that may be required before the examination begins.

Autolysis

For a post-mortem examination to be useful the bird must still be in a fresh state. Once the bird dies, the tissues will become stale and the enzymes contained in each cell will begin the process that breaks down the body. This is called autolysis. The smaller the bird and the longer it has been dead, the more likely it will be that autolysis has begun. This can markedly reduce the value of the post-mortem. The onset of autolysis can be delayed by thoroughly soaking the bird in soapy water, then wrapping the body in Glad Wrap™ or similar. Keep the bird chilled in the refrigerator, not the freezer, until the examination can be performed. Chilling allows a useful examination to be carried out up to 72 hours after death. It is most important not to freeze the bird unless it cannot be examined within 72 hours of death.

If you take the bird to your veterinarian for a post-mortem examination, it is preferable to take a bird that is still alive or one that has only recently died.

Equipment

Always use a face mask, gloves and have a set of instruments that are only used for avian post-mortem examination. I use the following instruments:
- Dispenser bottle containing disinfectant.
- Adson Rat-tooth forceps.
- 15cm sharp-tipped scissors.
- Iris scissors.
- Large utility scissors, for cutting larger bones.
- Sterile swabs and transport media.
- Microscope slides and coverslips.
- Buffered 10% Formalin™ and suitable range of containers.
- Sterile containers.
- 35mm camera with flash unit.

It is important to be aware of zoonoses, (diseases that pass from animals to people) and take steps to minimise the risk of these diseases being transmitted to yourself and others.

Inhalation of pathogens is a definite

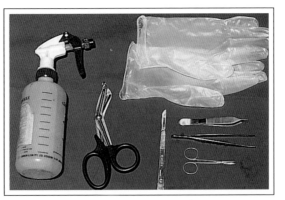

Post-mortem equipment – gloves, scissors, forceps, scalpel and spray bottle to wet the bird thoroughly.

risk, particularly with Psittacosis. To avoid inhaling disease particles follow these steps:

1. Thoroughly wet the cadaver with a detergent-based disinfectant, such as alcohol or Hibiclens™.
2. Wear a face mask.
3. Be aware of the pattern of airflow in the area the examination is being conducted. Stand with the airflow coming from behind you so that it flows across the cadaver and away.
4. The most dangerous time for inhalation is immediately after the abdominal cavity is opened and the sternum removed. There is a fine cloud of contaminated air that rises towards the dissector. This can be overcome by wetting the cadaver. An alternative is to temporarily cover the bird with a wet cloth during the opening procedure. This helps to trap the cloud.

External Examination

Before dissection is begun, a complete external examination should be performed. The bird should also be weighed.

Examine for any:
- Discharges (eyes, nostrils, beak, ears).
- Vomitus.
- Fractures (old or new).
- Wounds, haemorrhage or bruising.
- Ectoparasites (lice and mites of feathers or skin).
- Swellings (tumours, abdominal region, joints).
- Soiling or pasting of the vent or surrounding feathers.
- Feather damage or barring.
- Condition of feet/claws.
- Condition of oral cavity.

Make an estimate of:
- Age.
- Species (if not known).
- Gender (if dimorphic).
- Nutritional status (assess its body condition).
- Hydration status (feel the breast muscles).

Internal Examination

The dissection must be a systematic examination of all the body systems, performed in an orderly routine that will guarantee nothing is missed. There are as many methods of dissection as there are people performing them. The examination should not stop when an obvious lesion is found. This may not be the main problem and other important problems may be missed.

I lay the bird on its back and wet it thoroughly. Then I pluck all the feathers on the front of the bird so that I can examine the skin more closely before I cut. The whole surface of the bird that is facing you is exposed from the vent to the base of the beak.

The initial incision is in the midline of the bird. It begins at the base of the keel bone and only penetrates the skin. The incision is continued towards the neck, to expose the pectoral muscles and then up along the front of the neck. You can now see the oesophagus and crop.

Once the crop is encountered, it is opened with the scissors, and this is continued up into the mouth. The bones at the side of the beak are cut and the beak is moved across to allow you to see fully into the mouth. If there is sign of upper respiratory disease, the sinuses are opened and any contents are swabbed for culture and sensitivity. Samples may also be taken from the crop, oesophagus etc if indicated.

Make two incisions along each side of the trachea (windpipe) down to the syrinx and look for any foreign body, discharges etc.

Once the above areas are fully examined, the abdomen is opened and the ribs are cut down the side so that the keel bone can be lifted up and laid to one side. Examine all the organs before moving anything. Push the organs slightly to one side and then to the other side and examine the air sacs. Any lesions or discharges can be collected for culture and sensitivity. Impression smears from air sacs may be indicated. A simple way to collect air sac membrane is to strip the material underneath the keel bone, once it has been removed.

The first organ to remove is the heart. Sever the attachments of the great vessels and lift the heart away. A blood smear from the heart contents may show blood parasites.

Once the heart is removed, the proventriculus can be grasped where it sits below the heart and cut with scissors. This is lifted out of the body and, by snipping the air sac membranes, all the gastrointestinal tract (GIT) and the liver can be removed as a whole. Continue to dissect down and cut through the skin at the vent to keep the cloaca intact. This is laid to one side and the remaining organs examined. The gonads, kidneys, and adrenal gland are examined and dissected out as a group.

Remove and examine one or both lungs. Look for any masses (abscesses, foreign bodies etc).

The organs around the base of the neck are now examined. Pay particular attention to the thyroid glands (especially in Budgerigars). The oesophagus should be opened as lesions of *Trichomonas* (Canker) may be present.

Now turn to the GIT as it was removed. Samples can be taken from the liver and spleen (impression smears, swabs). Open the GIT beginning at the proventriculus, continuing down to the gizzard (ventriculus). Pay attention to the consistency of the tissues. Peel away the lining from the interior of the gizzard and examine for parasites underneath. Perform a scraping of the lining of the intestine in at least three separate positions. Examine smears of this material microscopically.

Remove the skin from the skull. Beware making conclusions about cranial haemorrhage based upon blood staining on the skull. This is a 'normal' change occuring after death as blood leaks from the tissues. Brain haemorrhage is suspected if there are blood clots or excessive collection of blood on, in or under the meninges (membranes on the surface of the brain).

It is not routine to remove the spinal cord. Open the major joints and look for any damage or inflammation of the surface of the joints and for any pus or other discharges. At the end of the dissection you should also have answered the following questions:
• Was the crop full or empty?
• Is there a blockage in the crop or proventriculus or any other part of the GIT?
• Was there normal grit in the gizzard?
• Are internal parasites a problem?
• Is the bird obese?
• Is the bird's reproductive system cycling as it should be?
• Do you suspect an infectious or non-infectious primary disease?
• Does the management of remaining birds need to be changed?

Histopathology

Histopathology is a useful tool where samples of tissues are sent to a pathologist who will microscopically examine them to detect minute changes in diseased tissue. Be aware that changes in organs seen during post-mortem examination are seldom pathognomonic (characteristic of a particular disease). Many obvious lesions can be misleading. With few exceptions, specimens should be carefully selected for further diagnostic tests, such as bacteriology or histopathology, to aid in a definitive diagnosis. Any sample intended for histopathology needs to be stored in greater than ten times its own volume in buffered 10% Formalin™.

Tissues routinely collected include lung, liver, spleen, proventriculus, gizzard, duodenum/pancreas, intestine, air sac membrane, kidney/gonad/adrenal glands, crop lining. They are usually all presented in a single container.

Clinical Pathology

The most useful diagnostic tests routinely performed are:

(a) Saline smears
  - intestinal wall scrapings for parasite eggs (usually select three separate sites along the small intestine).
  - faecal smears.
  - crop washes for *Trichomonas*.

(b) Impression smears of air sacs or organs (liver, spleen, obvious lesions).
  - Gram stain (bacteria, yeasts).
  - Macchiavello/MZN/Gimenez (*Chlamydophila psittaci*).
  - Diff Quik (cytology).

(c) Bacterial culture and sensitivity of swabs from heart blood, tissues, body fluids or intestinal/crop contents.

(d) Faecal flotation.

Most other clinical pathology tests should be carried out by an experienced avian pathologist. These tests will often give a definite diagnosis that is not available from most veterinary hospitals.

Toxicology Samples

Submit frozen tissues. For lead and zinc – collect liver and kidney stored in plastic bags. For chlorinated hydrocarbon – collect brain, liver, muscle and body fat wrapped in aluminium foil.

Post-mortem examination is one area of avian medicine that is under-serviced and under-utilised at present. It is a vital part of any aviary management program. A methodical approach combined with good records will enable you, working in conjunction with your avian veterinarian, to eliminate many of the problems that are a direct result of keeping birds in captivity.

ANTIBIOTICS IN AVICULTURE

We have all used antibiotics for ourselves and our birds. In fact, antibiotics are probably the most commonly used drugs in aviculture. There is a lot of confusion about the correct and best way to use them.

Incorrect usage can result in, at best, the drug not working or at worst, resistance to the antibiotic developing. The development of resistance is a very large problem because it means that antibiotics may be of no use if an infection breaks out in your aviary.

When you use an antibiotic, your aim is for the bird to develop strong, adequate levels of the drug in the bloodstream. Once this is achieved, it will be carried to the part of the body which is infected. The two most common causes of antibiotic failure are: If you use too low a dose of the antibiotic or if the dose is not being taken often enough, you will not achieve adequate levels in the bloodstream. If this happens, the infection will not be controlled and the bird may die. However, if you use an antibiotic incorrectly, you also risk developing resistance. In the long term this means putting other birds in the aviary at risk.

What is an Antibiotic?

Most people would say that an antibiotic is a drug we use to fight infection. In fact, many antibiotics are copies of chemicals that fungi naturally produce to protect themselves from attack by bacteria. To use antibiotics successfully you need to know a little more about them.

We can divide antibiotics into two broad groups as this will affect the way we use them.

- **Bacteriocidal** – these are the ones that destroy organisms. Because they actually kill, they are very effective in controlling infection. A well-known example is the Penicillin group (Amoxil™, Clavulox™, Pipril™).
- **Bacteriostatic** – these only inhibit growth and reproduction of organisms. These are not lethal, but have a contraceptive effect. The bird has to use its body defence system to kill the organisms. If the bird is very ill, it may not be able to do this. The major problem with this group is that once the antibiotic is ceased any organisms still alive can begin to reproduce again.

The sad news is that many of the common antibiotics suited for use in birds belong to the second group. Common examples are tetracyclines such as Terramycin™, Aureomycin™, Tricon™, Psittavet™.

Which Antibiotic Should I Use?

There are several types of infections that affect birds. Viruses, fungi, yeasts, protozoa, chlamydophila and bacteria are the most common. To know which antibiotic will work best in each situation, you have to know the cause each time. Viruses are not affected by any antibiotics. Fungi, yeasts, protozoa and chlamydophila each have their own special type of antibiotic. Bacteria have variable responses to each antibiotic which can change during a course of treatment if resistance develops.

It is easy to see that the answer to which antibiotic to use is to find the cause. In some cases finding the cause is easy, but in other cases it can be very difficult. For example, diarrhoea caused by worms or *Coccidia* can look the same as that caused by many bacteria. If you just choose an antibiotic and it does not help, it means your best guess was wrong. But was it wrong because you used an antibiotic that the bacteria was resistant to, or because the bird did not drink enough of the medicated water, or because the way you used it was wrong, or because the cause was not bacterial but fungal? The simple answer is that there are many reasons for antibiotic failure. Unfortunately, there is no such drug as the 'best antibiotic' that will work in all situations.

How do you identify the cause of

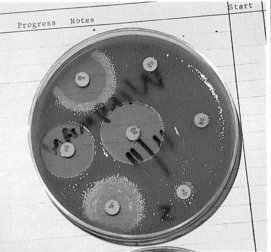

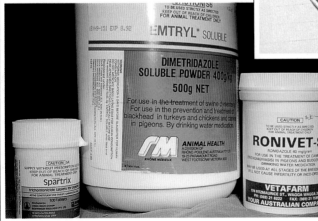

Above: Bacteriology plate showing the antibiotic sensitivity. The best antibiotic to use is the ones which leave a clear ring around the antibiotic disk. This is how we choose which drug will work best in a difficult situation. Left: Various antibiotics used in avian medication.

the problem? You need to run some laboratory tests on an individual bird, on samples of droppings etc. An alternative is to use your knowledge of diseases seen in your aviaries in the past and of successful treatments. Hence the importance of having post-mortems done on all birds that die. There is no substitute for knowing the facts of what went wrong.

There are some instances where the cause of a problem is easily identified and the choice of drugs is clear. For example, Emtryl™ (metronidazole) or Ronivet™ (ronidazole) is used for *Trichomonas* (Canker), Mycostatin™ (nystatin) is used for fungi and yeasts especially *Candida* and Baycox™ (toltrazuril) or Coccivet™ (amprolium) is used for Coccidiosis.

If the wrong drug is used in the above cases, failure is likely to occur.

When the cause of infection is bacteria, the choice of drug is not so clear. Many bacteria vary in their resistance to each different antibiotic. The ideal is to identify the bacteria in a laboratory and find which antibiotic will affect it, using a so-called culture and sensitivity test. This is not always possible for economic reasons or lack of time. Often veterinarians make an educated guess based on past experiences.

Bacterial resistance to an antibiotic can be increased by either overuse (using the same antibiotics on every sick bird) or underuse (using the antibiotic at too low a dose or for too short a time, eg one day each week).

It is most important that an antibiotic be used at the correct dose for the correct period of time. This will vary with the type of antibiotic and the way it is used. You should know this for every antibiotic you use.

Many of the potent antibiotics need to be given by injection to be reliable. I think injection is a must in a critically ill bird as this gives high blood levels quickly. Most sick birds will show improvement more quickly if they are given an injection of antibiotics at the beginning of their disease. The ideal would be to continue with regular injections until the bird is fully recovered. In many cases this cannot be maintained and the bird is then treated with medication in-water or directly to the beak.

Why do Birds become Infected?

This is a difficult question to answer in specific cases. Stress plays a major role by decreasing the bird's natural immunity and an infectious agent which otherwise would be controlled, grasps the opportunity.

Every day birds are exposed to potential infection from microorganisms on your hands and clothes, in their food and water and nearly every part of their environment. Poor nutrition, an unbalanced diet and an unhygienic environment can increase the risk of problems developing.

Once an infection is underway the signs the bird shows will depend upon the organs affected. Most birds just look sick – fluffed up, eyes closed, heavy breathing etc. They lose body salts and fluids by vomiting, diarrhoea and even by just breathing. They burn up body protein and fats to maintain their body temperature. Usually none of this is replaced because sick birds will not eat or drink very much.

All sick birds need fluids (water), body salts (electrolytes) and a source of protein and energy as well as any drugs to treat an infection. Many birds are in a critical stage before the early signs of illness are recognised, because they are experts at hiding these signs.

Rules for Using Antibiotics in Birds

1. Keep handling to a minimum to avoid stress. Have everything prepared before you catch the bird.
2. Medication in-water is useful to treat a flock or large aviary collection, but is not as reliable with individual birds.
3. With in-water medication, the dose you give the bird will vary with changes in water consumption. Be careful in hot weather or if parents are feeding young birds, as it is easy to overdose, particularly with Emtryl™. Be careful with providing other water

sources that allow the bird to drink less from the water dish. Soaked seed, greens, fruit or other foods containing moisture will cause the bird to drink less water and so take in less medication.

4. For in-water medications avoid using a container that will interfere with the medication. In particular, avoid galvanised metal bowls and earthenware dishes. The best containers are either glass or stainless steel. Place the container in the shade. Exposure to light and heat causes the medication to lose strength. Most antibiotic solutions should be made freshly each day. The ideal is to make them up in the evening and place them in the aviary at this time. This allows the birds to have a drink in the evening and again in the morning. The cool and dark of night causes less deterioration of the medication than occurs during the day.

5. All antibiotics can reduce normal bowel bacteria. Many of these bacteria produce some of the essential vitamins. These bacteria may need to be replaced, eg yoghurt or probiotic. As well, give a vitamin supplement and a small amount of grit to overcome any losses.

6. Injections are often necessary in preference to drugs given in food or water because some drugs are poorly absorbed from the gut. Other drugs that would be normally well absorbed may be decreased if food is present or if there is damage to the gut lining from disease, parasites or nutritional deficiency.

Dosages of Antibiotics

Many of the doses recommended today are based upon what has worked in the past. There is research being done at the moment to establish more specific dosages. Birds generally need higher doses than mammals. There is a large variation in the ability of different species of birds to absorb, use and excrete the same antibiotic. Eventually there will be doses recommended for each species. A lower dose is needed if given by injection compared to administering in-food or in-water.

Methods of Administering Antibiotics

In-water

This is acceptable for treating large numbers of birds or for wild birds where handling is not desirable. It may also be useful for some gut infections where the drug does not need to be absorbed. Because the bird only takes small amounts at a time or takes less than is required, there is an increased chance of resistance developing. Many sick birds will not drink enough or will reject the water because of colour or taste.

Some drugs, particularly tetracyclines, rapidly lose their strength in water and need to be replaced 2–3 times a day. All antibiotics should be replaced daily. Avoid exposure to direct sunlight. Use glass containers rather than plastic or metal, other than stainless steel.

In-food

This is useful if the bird has a favourite food or one that is easy to eat, eg crushed apple or banana, soaked seed, corn mash, peanut butter, boiled rice etc. Some birds will refuse to eat or are too weak to eat. Some drugs are inactivated by food, eg chloramphenicol and tetracyclines (inactivated by calcium).

Oral Medication

This refers to medication given into the mouth or crop from an eye dropper, syringe, feeding tube or crop needle. Some oral suspensions are flavoured and birds will readily take them, eg Amoxil™ drops seem to be accepted better than Clavulox™ drops.

Do not give the medication too rapidly or it will come out the nostrils, frightening the bird and making subsequent treatment difficult. Many of these medications are water soluble and will easily mix with food. As with medication in food and water, absorption may be erratic.

Injections

This allows the exact dose to be given efficiently. This is the best way to give drugs that are poorly absorbed from the gut, eg gentamicin, chloramphenicol.

It can be quite stressful as the bird has to be caught. This must be balanced against the more rapid absorption and the more effective drugs that can be used this way.

Injections are usually given into the breast muscle. Some drugs are very irritant if injected into a muscle and must be injected directly into a vein.

With injecting into a muscle the site must be varied each time or the muscle will be damaged. The most common way to do this is to use alternate sides of the breast muscle, and vary top to bottom with subsequent injections. (Refer to *How to Give an Injection* on page 32).

Topical Medication

Antibiotic and antifungal agents can be applied directly onto the skin or into the eye. Creams and ointments must be used with care as the oily component can damage feathers. Water-based sprays or water soluble powders are preferred.

Nebulisation

Deep respiratory or air sac infections are occasionally treated by antibiotics in a fog from a nebuliser. This is used to penetrate the thick pus contained deep in the lungs and air sacs, as normal treatment cannot reach these areas. The equipment can be expensive and the treatment must be carried out for a long time, sometimes from weeks to months.

Why Antibiotics can Fail in Birds

In most cases the specific type of bacteria causing an infection is not known and an educated guess is made as to which drug should be used. There is not always time to wait until tests can demonstrate the cause. Experience becomes the best guide.

Occasionally, with very resistant bacteria, the best drug will harm the patient, eg gentamicin can cause kidney damage. This is a risk that is only worthwhile for severe illness. In this case, a better choice would be Amikacin™ which is less toxic but a closely related drug.

The bird may not take an adequate amount of the medication if it is given in food or water. How does this happen? The bird refuses to eat the medicated food or water because of colour or taste. The presence of food, milk, calcium etc, interferes with absorption from the gut. Similarly, disease, parasites (worms, *Coccidia*, protozoa) or vitamin deficiency can interfere with absorption, so that although the dose given to the bird is correct, not enough reaches the bloodstream.

If the bird has a low level of immunity, it will not be able to take advantage of the drug as it is not strong enough to cure itself. The bird will die, not because the drug was incorrect, but because the disease has advanced so far that the body was unable to carry out the normal healing processes.

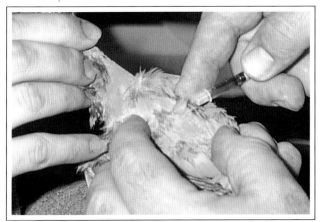

Some antibiotics need to be given for a long time to be successful. For example, tetracyclines when used for Psittacosis, must be used for 30–45 days. If used for less time the bird will initially appear to be cured but will soon relapse and become ill again.

Intramuscular injection being administered.

Some organisms can never be totally eliminated from the body. Treatment reduces them to a level the body can cope with. This is seen in some cases of Salmonellosis and Psittacosis. The bird recovers with treatment, but the disease will recur if the bird is stressed.

Antibiotics Commonly used in Aviculture

Bacteriocidal	Bacteriostatic
Cephalosporins	Chloramphenicol
Aminoglycosides	Erythromycin
Quinolones	Lincomycin
Penicillins	Lincomycin and Spectinomycin
Nystatin	Nitrofurans
	Sulphonamides
	Sulphonamides and Trimethoprim
	Tetracyclines
	Tylosin

Anti-yeast Medications Commonly used in Aviculture

Ketoconazole
Nystatin
Flucytosine
Chlorhexidine
Itraconazole
Fluconazole

Antibiotics most Commonly used for Gram negative Infections

Enrofloxacin
Amikacin
Third Generation Cephalosporins
Piperacillin
Trimethoprim and Sulphonamides

AVIAN PARASITE CONTROL

The most common complication of captivity is the increased exposure to parasite burdens. When I am asked for 'something to worm my birds', a little time spent discussing history, species and the type of aviary helps me to select the most effective treatment as well as good practical advice regarding administration. It is important to realise that controlling worms is not just a matter of 'giving them the right wormer'. It is better to use drugs as part of a program that helps prevent the birds coming into contact with worm eggs or the intermediate host that carries the worms.

Any advice given should aim towards prevention rather than just regular treatment. There is a wide variety of species as well as many and varied conditions under which birds are housed. The type and design of an aviary can be a significant help in controlling the survival of worm eggs.

Hairworm *(Capillaria)*

Signs:
- Diarrhoea (with or without blood).
- Weight loss.
- Depression.
- Not eating.
- Vomiting.
- Anaemia.

The *Capillaria* are parasites that live in the lining of the bird's intestine, crop or oesophagus. They damage the lining of these areas and may cause haemorrhage. Birds are unable to absorb nutrients from their food. This can eventually lead to death.

This worm is passed between birds by eating another bird's droppings containing the *Capillaria* eggs. The eggs can live in the ground for several months and then pass onto another bird.

Diagnosis is by examining the droppings under a microscope and identifying the characteristic eggs. The worms are quite fine (like a cotton thread) and easily missed on a post-mortem examination.

These worms can be difficult to treat. In one situation they will be removed by a wormer but not in the next. You may need to try several wormers to remove them successfully. Recommended treatments are levamisole (Nilverm™, Avitrol™), oxfendazole (Benzelmin™, Synanthic™, Systamex™) and fenbendazole (Panacur 25™).

A common problem in Budgerigars, macaws, conures, African Lovebirds, pigeons, gallinaceous birds (pheasants, quail, peafowl, partridge etc), canaries, weavers, whydahs, jays, mynahs and honey-eaters.

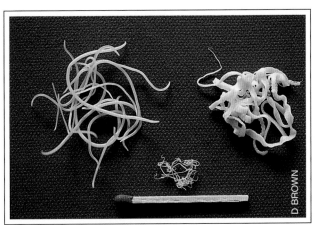

Roundworm *(Ascaridia)*

Signs:
- Chronic weight loss.
- Diarrhoea.
- Weakness.
- Depression.
- Poor growth of young birds.

Above: Worms. Top right Tapeworm, top left Roundworm, bottom Gizzardworm. Below: Roundworms sitting inside the intestine of a lovebird.

These worms are the most common parasite found in birds that spend a significant amount of time on the ground and come in contact with their droppings.

This worm is passed between birds by eating another bird's droppings containing the roundworm eggs. The eggs can live in the ground, provided there are moist conditions, for several

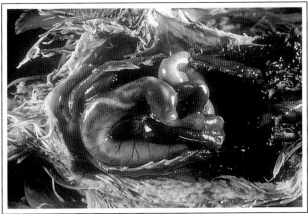

months and then pass onto another bird. In dry conditions the eggs die quickly.

Once the eggs are inside the bird, they hatch and the juvenile worms live close to the lining of the intestine. They cause irritation and interfere with the bird's ability to absorb nutrients. In the right conditions, the birds will take in large numbers of eggs and they all hatch at once, causing a blockage, leading to death.

Some of these worms can be shared by parrots, pigeons and gallinaceous birds, so if they are sharing an aviary you need to worm them all quite regularly.

This is a common problem in Australian parrots particularly Budgerigars, Cockatiels, the *Polytelis* genus (Princess, Regent and Superb Parrots), the *Neophema* genus (Scarlet-chested, Turquoise, Bourke's, Elegant, Blue-winged, Rock and Orange-bellied Parrots), the *Psephotus* genus (Red-rumped, Mulga, Golden-shouldered, Hooded and Blue-bonnet Parrots) and rosellas. Roundworms are uncommon in passerines (canaries and finches).

Prevention is best achieved by having a dry, well-drained floor and removing all the droppings once a week. Concrete floors or wire floors are very successful in controlling worms. Birds in these enclosures need worming once to twice a year. Birds kept in aviaries with dirt floors need to be wormed at least every three months. To monitor how effective your worming program is you should have the droppings tested one week after you have wormed the birds.

The most useful drugs for controlling roundworms are: ivermectin (Ivomec™), moxidectin (Cydectin™), levamisole (Nilverm™, Avitrol™), oxfendazole (Benzelmin™, Synanthic™, Systamex™) and fenbendazole (Panacur 25™).

Tapeworms

Signs:
- Mucous in droppings.
- Tapeworm segments in the droppings.
- Weight loss.
- Sudden death.

The tapeworm and gizzardworm are carried by many small insects. When the birds eat the insects they take in the eggs of the tapeworm or gizzardworm. For this reason these worms are mainly a problem in birds which eat a lot of insects, mainly in finches and occasionally in cockatoos (particularly if wild caught), Eclectus and African Grey Parrots.

Tapeworms cause problems as they interfere with the absorption of nutrients in the intestines. If they build up to large numbers, they can cause an obstruction in the intestines. In insectivorous finches these worms are a common cause of death – particularly Diamond Firetails and Parrot Finches.

The tapeworm is not a problem in small numbers, but it can build up if the conditions are right – humid conditions and plenty of safe hiding places as well as a good food source for the insects. The practice of having a compost heap or colony of mealworms on the floor of the aviary helps keep these worms present.

Tests on the droppings that will detect other worms often will not detect tapeworms. They can be difficult to diagnose. Often a course of praziquantel (Droncit™, Avitrol Plus™, Wormout™ tablets and gel, Prazivet™, Prazilev™, Tape Out Powder™) or oxfendazole (Benzelmin™, Synanthic™, Systamex™) is given if you suspect the birds may have tapeworm. To prevent tapeworm problems use the following techniques. Regularly clean up your aviaries and use 'safe' insecticide sprays (eg Coopex™), feed your birds alternatives to insects such as egg and biscuit mix, commercial diets, cheese, or insectivore mixes.

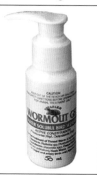

Wormout™ Tablets and Gel.

Gizzardworm is a problem in finches and not

parrots. In Australian aviaries it is a common cause of death in both native and exotic finches. This worm lives under the hard lining of the gizzard. The damage it causes to the gizzard causes problems with grinding and digesting the seeds. Many birds will pass whole seeds in their droppings. This worm passes characteristic eggs that can be detected with standard laboratory examination (faecal flotation) of the droppings. This can be a difficult worm to remove. Successful treatment has been achieved with levamisole (Nilverm™, Avitrol™) or oxfendazole (Benzelmin™, Synanthic™, Systamex™) or moxidectin (Cydectin™).

Type of Aviary

The aviary structure, particularly the floor, will determine the survival rate of parasite eggs or the intermediate hosts. Areas of concern are:

- Areas that are consistently moist provide a suitable environment for long-term egg survival, eg poor drainage of floors, water bowl overflow area and dark or shaded areas that never dry out fully.
- Dishes, food bowls etc on the ground provide suitable housing for insects. Some aviculturists who regularly feed insects, such as mealworms, encourage them to set up a colony on the floor of the aviary. The mealworms are exposed to the resident birds' faeces and can help the worms to survive and be passed onto your birds.
- Wooden frames of aviaries encourage more insects such as mites, cockroaches etc, more so than metal frames, as they have more cracks for insects to hide in.
- Dirt floors allow more eggs to survive than do solid floors such as concrete. A little sand spread over a concrete floor helps to keep the floor dry and makes it easier to sweep and keep clean.
- Pay particular attention to areas where birds spend a lot of time, especially around food and water dishes or nesting boxes. These areas must be kept clean and dry. The heavy traffic in these areas allows the build-up of large numbers of eggs and makes it more likely for eggs to be passed onto the birds. You must have very good drainage around all water bowls so that there is not a constant patch of moisture on the floor next to the dish.
- Perches should never be positioned above food or water dishes as this encourages the droppings to be eaten when they contaminate the food or water. Perches should be replaced regularly, as soon as they show signs of a build-up of droppings.
- Floors that make it harder for birds to come into contact with their droppings can be a very effective way of controlling worms. An example is the wire floor of suspended aviaries. You can use your imagination to apply this principle in other ways.

Administration of Worming Drugs

This is a difficult problem for some species. It is always a compromise between the easiest way for the aviculturist and the most efficacious way for the birds. The choices available are basically the same as other animals.

Oral

- **Tablets**

  Are suitable for straight-billed birds such as pigeons, quail and pheasants. Not successful for administration to hook-billed birds such as parrots or small birds such as finches.

- **Drops**

  When administering, beware of inhalation. This is not an accurate method as birds can flick the medication out of their mouth so you are unsure how much is given.

- **Gavage (Crop) needle**

  This is my preferred means of worming most birds. Using a syringe with a crop needle attached allows you to measure any medication accurately. You know that the bird has had the correct dose. Delivering the medication directly into the bird's crop avoids any problems with inhaling the medication. The handler does not need to be more skilled than with some of the other methods. It is a skill that anyone, who can chew gum and walk a straight line, can easily learn. This technique often worries beginners. My advice is that every aviculturist MUST have this skill. Find a friend who is experienced and have them walk you through this technique, as it is a powerful tool for saving birds' lives.

- **In-food medication**
  Consider the flavour of the drug administered. For example, Ivomec™ is quite bitter, Panacur™ is pleasant tasting and Benzelmin™ is both odourless and tasteless. Use highly flavoured and attractive food supplements such as cake, apple and any favoured food items.
- **In-water medication**
  This method is not suitable for desert species which can overconsume as they drink large amounts of water twice daily rather than small amounts throughout the day. Placing coloured or bitter medications in water can cause birds to become suspicious of the water and avoid it. I have known colonies of finches that became dehydrated three days after their water was medicated with a bitter wormer, as they refused to drink from the water bowl, even when refilled with fresh water.

Topical
This is a quick and simple method, although there are not many suitable drugs available at present. The most common treatment available is Ivomec™ applied as drops to the back of the neck for parasite control.

Parenteral Injection
Subcutaneous and intramuscular injections are not very popular due to the delicacy of administration.

Summary of Administration of Worming Drugs
Some examples of commonly used parasite treatments include:
- **Drops into the beak:** Panacur 25™, Avitrol™, Avitrol Plus™, Ivomec™, Cydectin™.
- **Gavage needle:** Panacur 25™, Cydectin™, Ivomec™, Nilverm™, Wormout ™ gel.
- **In-feed:** Nilverm™, Synanthic™, Benzelmin™, Panacur 25™, Valbazen™.
- **In-water:** Nilverm™, Ivomec™, Cydectin™, Wormout™ gel, Avitrol™, Avitrol Plus™, Prazivet™.
- **Tablets:** Vital™, Avitrol™, Wormout™.

Parasite Prevention
Strategic Drenching
This is an important consideration. It is much better to plan and anticipate the most effective time to worm your birds. It is better to identify when the birds are more likely to be affected by the worms and to treat them at that time rather than do it at set intervals or when you just happen to remember that it has been a while since you last wormed them. This will save the life of many birds. These times are:
- Prior to the breeding season. This helps reduce parasites being passed onto the young.
- After heavy rains or a period of steady rain, when the aviary floor is wet.
- During warm temperatures, particularly when the humidity is high.
- During times of stress.
- When a bird is brought home for the first time. As part of your quarantine process, treat all birds at least twice before you release them into the aviary.

You can identify the parasites that are causing your birds a problem by having your veterinarian examine the droppings under a microscope. This helps determine the best wormer to use and monitors whether the current wormer is really working effectively. Repeat this examination of the droppings at least twice a year. In addition, any bird that dies should be opened and examined for the presence of any parasites as a monitor of the situation in your aviary – this is something you can learn to do yourself.

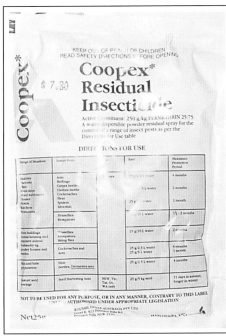

Coopex Insecticide™ sachet.

Control Intermediate Hosts
- Use 'safe' insecticides eg Coopex™ to clean up any possible intermediate hosts that inhabit the floor, cracks in the walls etc.
- Regularly treat or remove perches, nesting boxes, food and water dishes. Place all dishes, boxes etc off the floor of the aviary.

Improve Aviary Design
- Consider the type of floor. People often ask which is the best floor substrate. It is not a matter of one floor substrate being better than another. Every floor substrate has its problems and all need to be cleaned regularly to remove food particles and droppings that are present. The trick is to understand the shortcomings of the floor substrate you are using and work out how to overcome any problems.

Concrete is more easily managed, as cleaning is easier. However, unless it is finished and smoothed with a metal float, the rough surface can trap remnants of food and droppings and pools of water will collect in depressions creating a medium for the growth of disease organisms. Blue metal or large stones provide good drainage but trap seed and can be difficult to clean effectively. Sand or dirt needs to be swept or raked at least once weekly so that the upper layer containing food and droppings is removed. Wire bottom cages are mandatory for some species such as lorikeets as their liquid droppings cling to everything – these should be hosed regularly to soften the build-up and then cleaned off with a jet of water.

The ease of cleaning needs to be balanced against the stress caused to the birds when you are cleaning inside the aviary. Visit other aviculturists and see how their substrate is managed, then look at your birds and aviaries and decide which substrate best suits your conditions.
- Pay attention to vermin proofing against wild birds, snakes, rats and mice etc.
- Remove any damp areas. Improve drainage. Don't hose out bowls onto the aviary floor.
- In high rainfall areas, a completely covered roof and a sun porch or walkway is recommended.

Common Parasiticides

The following are commonly used parasiticides. Be aware that they are usually not registered for use in this manner or in the species you are treating. For this reason the doses and recommendations listed here are subject to the consideration that all persons using these drugs do so entirely at their own risk.

Many of the worming medications have different doses for parrots, finches, pigeons or other species. Always carefully check the dose for your species and measure quantities accurately.

Levamisole

Levamisole is a good choice for flock treatment of most worms except tapeworm. It has a bitter taste. Remove water from the aviary for 12 hours before administering. Add Glucodin™, honey or sugar for flavouring.

***Avitrol*™ syrup** (levamisole 10mg/ml)
- ***Finches:*** Use 0.1ml per 40 gram body weight for larger finches (ie Zebra Finch) for 3 days. Use 0.05ml per 20 gram body weight for smaller finches (ie Orange-breasted Finch) for 3 days.

***Avitrol Plus*™ syrup** (levamisole 10mg/ml + praziquantel 2mg/ml)
- **Dose:** Can be given directly into the beak at a dose of 1 drop per 10 gram body weight. In the drinking water it is used at a dose of 0.5ml (12 drops) in 20ml water or 25ml per litre of water.

Doses for Avitrol™ and Avitrol Plus™ syrups		
Species	**Body weight**	**Number of Drops**
Finch	15 gram	1
Finch	30 gram	3
Budgerigar	50 gram	5
Cockatiel	80 gram	8
Cockatoo	500 gram	50

***Avitrol*™ tablets** (levamisole 20mg) and ***Avitrol Plus*™ tablets** (levamisole 20mg + praziquantel 4mg)
- **Dose:** Use 1/2 a tablet per 250–500 gram body weight; 1 tablet for 500–750 gram body weight; 1 1/2 tablets for 750–1000 gram body weight.

Do not feed birds before or 3 hours after treatment. Treatment during the breeding season or racing season (pigeons) is not recommended. Vomiting may occur. To reduce the likelihood of vomiting do not handle birds for at least 10 minutes after treatment.

***Avitrol*™ syrup** and **tablets** are used for the treatment of threadworm (*Capillaria* sp), caecal worm (*Heterakis* sp), roundworm (*Ascaridia* sp), gape worm (*Syngamus* sp), gizzardworm (*Acuaria* sp).

***Avitrol Plus*™ syrup** and **tablets** are used for the treatment of threadworm (*Capillaria* sp), caecal worm (*Heterakis* sp), roundworm (*Ascaridia* sp), gape worm (*Syngamus* sp), gizzardworm (*Acuaria* sp) and tapeworms (*Choanotaenia* sp and *Raillietinia* sp).

Parrots appear to be less tolerant than pigeons to levamisole. Do not dose in extremely hot, dry weather or treat stressed birds, or birds that are feeding young.

***L-Spartakon*™ tablets** (20mg) **Dose:** Use one tablet per 500 gram body weight.

***Nilverm Injection*™** (89mg/ml)
- **Dose:** Use 8ml per litre of water.

***Nilverm Oral Drench*™** (32mg/ml) **Dose:** Use 25ml per litre of water.

***Nilverm Oral LV*™** (80mg/ml)
- **Dose:** Use 9ml per litre of water.
- ***Parrots:*** Can be given by crop needle directly into the crop. Mix it with water in a 1:1 ratio (eg 5ml water with 5ml Nilverm Oral LV™) and give 0.1ml per 100 gram body weight for 3 consecutive days. Do not inject any liquid into the crop unless you are confident that the crop tube is correctly placed.

***Nilverm Pig & Poultry Wormer*™** (16mg/ml)
- **Dose:** Use 50ml per litre of water.
- ***Finches:*** Use 40ml per litre of drinking water for 24 hours. Repeat one day a week for a total of four weeks.
- ***Parrot Finches:*** Use a half dose (20ml per litre of water). Repeat one day a week for a total of four weeks.

***Vital*™ tablets** (20mg) **Dose:** Use 1 tablet per 500 gram body weight.

Fenbendazole

This is a suspension, so it will settle if used as in-water medication.

Panacur 25™ (25mg/ml)

This is best given by crop needle but most birds do not mind the taste so it can be mixed with soft food or smeared over fruit etc.

- **In-food dose:** Mix 8ml Panacur 25™ with 12ml cooking/vegetable oil in 1kg of bird seed. Use this as sole source of food for one week and repeat in one month.
- **Crop needle or oral dose:** Use 0.1–0.2ml per 50 gram body weight for 3 days consecutively.
- **Nectar mix:** Mix 8ml Panacur 25™ in 1 litre of nectar. Provide this at normal volume of nectar for 6 days as the only nectar supplement. Provide fresh nectar every 24 hours. Take similar precautions as with normal nectar, providing only the volume that the birds will consume quickly, as nectar that is sitting around on a warm day can deteriorate and become contaminated with dangerous bacteria.

Panacur 100™ (100mg/ml)

Not recommended even if diluted to above dose. Fatalities have been recorded with this preparation.

Oxfendazole

This is similar to Panacur 25™ in action. When used as an in-water medication, the mixture should be provided fresh every 24 hours. This drug comes in three forms – Synanthic™, Systamex™ and Benzelmin™.

Synanthic™ (18.12g/L)

- ***Finches:*** Use 25ml per litre of water in a shallow dish for 3 days. Make fresh daily.
- ***Aviary recipe* (finches, softbills, pigeons):** Mix 12ml with 10ml vegetable oil to form an emulsion. Mix this well through the seed and allow it to stand for 12 hours. Use this as the only source of food for 5 days. Provide a fresh source of seed every 24 hours. Make fresh daily.

Systamex™ (90.6g/L)

- ***Finches:*** Use 5ml per litre of water for 3 days. Make fresh daily.
- ***Parrots:*** Dilute 1ml with 20ml of water and administer 0.25ml per 100 gram body weight by crop needle for 3–5 days. Make fresh daily.

Benzelmin™ (200g/L)

- ***Finches:*** Use 2.2ml/L of water for 3 days. Make fresh daily.
- ***Parrots:*** Dilute 1ml with 50ml of water and then give 0.25ml per 100 gram body weight by crop needle for 3–5 days. Make fresh daily.

Albendazole

Valbazen™ (113mg/ml)

- ***Finches:*** Administer in-water 5ml per litre of water for 3 days. Make fresh every 24 hours. Offer clear water for 2 days then repeat.
- ***Direct to the beak:*** Give 0.05ml (approximately 1 drop) per 100 gram body weight once daily for 3 days or 0.1ml per 100 gram body weight as a single dose.

This product is related to Panacur 25™ and Synanthic™ so it can be used in similar circumstances. It has been used to treat resistant forms of *Capillaria* with some success.

Ivermectin

These drugs are effective against quite a few worms including *Ascaridia,* some *Capillaria* and some *Acuaria* worms, but are not useful for any tapeworms. All forms of Ivomec™ are also very effective for Scaly-face Mite and Scaly-leg Mite in Budgerigars, Kakarikis and Neophema Grass Parrots.

Ivomec Liquid for Sheep™ (0.8g/L)

This sheep drench is used without diluting in water and administered by crop needle. It is a water-based product, not suitable for penetrating the skin. The application as a spot-on on the back of the neck was suitable for the discontinued Avomec™ and for the more recent Ivomec Spotton™ skin application, but is not suitable for Ivomec Liquid for Sheep™.

- **Dose:** Administer 0.1ml per 100 gram body weight by crop needle. It can also be mixed in drinking water at 15–20ml per litre. The product is stable in water for approximately 12 hours so it needs to be provided fresh twice daily.

Ivomec RV for Sheep™ (2.0g/L)

This new product is 2.5 times stronger than Ivomec Liquid for Sheep™, which is the only product that is safe to deliver undiluted to the beak. Ivomec RV for Sheep™ must be diluted or used only on large birds.

Ivomec Pour-on for Cattle™ (5g/L)

This product is suitable for penetrating the skin, being designed to penetrate cattle skin. It has been used in a range of birds. The medication is applied to an area of bare skin, usually on the back of the neck. This product is

Dose of Ivomec Pour-on for Cattle™ as drops on bare skin.	
Species	Number of Drops
Finch	1
Canary	2
Neophema	4
Rosella	8
Cockatoo	20

approximately six times as strong as Ivomec Liquid for Sheep™, so only a small amount is required.

- **Dose:** Apply 0.015ml per 100 gram body weight. Alternately dilute 1ml with 9ml of propylene glycol and use 0.15ml per 100 gram body weight.

Ivomec Antiparasitic Injection for Cattle™ (10g/L)

It is not recommended to mix this product in water as it is not soluble. Deaths have been reported by injecting Ivormec™ in some finches.

- **Parrots:** Dilute 1:100 with propylene glycol and give 0.2ml per 100 gram body weight by crop needle.

Moxidectin

Cydectin™ (100mcg/ml)

Trials are still being conducted to confirm the correct dose. The current dose being used is 0.2ml per 100 gram body weight by crop needle. If placed directly into the beak it often causes vomiting. Beware of the solution contacting human eyes or skin as it is quite irritant. Do not mix with other worming drugs. This product is reported to be effective for *Capillaria*, roundworm, Scaly-face mites and Air Sac mites. Avoid contamination of creeks and dams when you are disposing of the product, as it can damage the insects and fish. Do not repeat dosing of this at less than six week intervals. It is considered to have a better safety margin than ivermectins.

For in-water medication, measure the water intake over 24 hours then calculate the amount of moxidectin based on the weight of the birds in that aviary. Place the amount of moxidectin in the drinking water they should drink over 24 hours. Offer the medicated water containing the calculated dose until all water is consumed. If you cannot measure the water intake, a commonly used flock dose for parrots is 20ml per litre of drinking water.

- **Pigeons:** Individual adult bird dose is 0.25ml into the mouth or crop. Flock dose is 5ml per litre of water for 24 hours.
- **Finches:** Individual dose is 0.1ml per 50 gram body weight into the crop. Flock dose is 5ml per litre of water for 3–5 days, made fresh daily.

As an in-water medication this product is more stable than ivermectin. It is not recommended to use the cattle preparation as its solvent is irritating to birds.

- **Parrots:** Individual dose is 0.2ml per 100 gram bodyweight by crop needle. Flock dose is 20ml per litre of drinking water.

Praziquantel
Droncit™

This product is for treating tapeworms only, although when mixed with other wormers, eg Avitrol Plus™ and Wormout™ gel, the medication treats a broad spectrum of worms.

The following medications have been used:

Droncit™ **cat tablet (23mg) or** *Droncit*™ **dog tablet (50mg)**

- *Finches:* Use 50mg per kg of seed. Crush the tablet and mix with a small amount of vegetable oil or cod liver oil. Mix through the seed. Feed fresh every day for 3 days.
- Estimate the total weight of finches in the aviary, eg 50 x 20 gram finches = 1000 grams. For each 1000 grams of finches use $1/2$ a 23mg tablet or $1/4$ of a 50mg tablet. Mix the crushed tablet evenly through their favourite soft food (cake, egg and biscuit, apple etc). Place this treated food in as many sites as possible throughout the aviary so that the dominant birds will not eat it all. Repeat in 10–14 days.
- *Parrots:* Crush 1 Droncit™ cat tablet (23mg) or $1/2$ Droncit™ dog tablet (50mg) and mix with 1.0ml water in a syringe. Give 0.1ml per 100 gram body weight, immediately the solution is mixed, before it begins to settle out.

The Droncit™ tablets are not water soluble and therefore are unsuitable for in-water medication.

Avitrol Plus™ **syrup** (levamisole 10mg/ml + praziquantel 2mg/ml): Give 1 drop per 10 gram body weight into the beak or 1ml per 20ml of drinking water for 24 hours.

Prazivet™ **solution** (25mg/ml): Use 5ml per litre of drinking water for 24 hours.

Wormout™ **tablets** (oxfendazole 20mg + praziquantel 20mg): Give 1 tablet per 2kg body weight.

Wormout™ **gel:** (oxfendazole 20g/L + praziquantel 20g/L): Use 1ml per 80ml of drinking water. Supply for 2 days. Individual bird dose is 0.05ml per100 gram bodyweight as a single dose. Repeat every 3 months.

The Droncit™ injectable solution has been withdrawn from the market.

Toltrazuril
Baycox™ (25g/L)

This is the most effective medication for controlling Coccidiosis. Do not use in galvanised or rusty iron water containers.

Coccidiosis is an emerging problem in the Budgerigar. It does not pass eggs (oocysts) that can be detected in the droppings until the birds are quite ill, and therefore can be difficult to detect. If you suspect that it is a problem in your Budgerigar flock, give them treatment for up to 5 days.

Ideally you should measure the amount of water the birds drink over an 8 hour period in a day and deliver this volume with the Baycox™. Then give the birds clear water for the remaining hours until they are medicated the next day. The aim is to provide the medication only over an 8 hour period each day.

- *Most birds:* 3ml per litre of drinking water for 3 days.
- *Pigeons:* 2ml per litre of drinking water for 2 days.
- *Budgerigars:* 3ml per litre of drinking water for 2–5 days.

Amprolium

This product will only control Coccidiosis, it has no activity against worms.

The following medications have been used:

Amprolmix Plus™ (amprolium 250g/kg + ethopabate 16g/kg)

- Week 1: 3ml per litre of water.
- Week 2: 2ml per litre of water.
- Week 3: 1ml per litre of water.

Then 1ml per litre of water for one week each month.

Coccivet™ (amprolium 80g/L + ethopabate 5.1g/L)
   Use 1.5ml per litre of drinking water for 5–7 days. Repeat as needed.
   Other formulations available (for doses follow manufacturer's directions):
Keystat Coccidiostat™ solution
Amprolium 200™
Amprosol™

Permethrin
Coopex™ (250g/kg)
   A synthetic pyrethrin insecticide for use in aviaries. Use Coopex™ as follows:
   This preparation is the subject of a pesticide order under the Pesticides and Chemicals Act 1978 that allows it to be legally used around aviaries. Before use read all the directions on the packet as well as the information specified in the pesticide order.
   This product can be used around the aviary to help control some of the insect intermediate hosts that will pass on tapeworms and *Acuaria*.
   For ants, flies, moths, mealworms, red mites and forage mites: a 25 gram sachet per 5 litres of water. Soak areas that may harbour mites and insects.
   For cockroaches: a 25 gram sachet per 2.5 litres of water.

Avian Insect Liquidator™
   For parrots, finches and canaries use a 5% solution. Mix 1 part concentrate made up to 20 parts total volume with water (add 1ml to 19ml water). Place solution in a spray pump. Hold the spray 30–40 cm from the birds and apply 4–5 sprays (3–4ml) to the bird. Also spray cages, aviaries, perches and nestboxes thoroughly with the diluted product. Repeat every 6 weeks or as required.

Summary of Worm Treatment
* Give some thought to which worms are the main problem in the species of birds in your aviary.
* Change your management and aviary design to help minimise exposure to worms or their intermediate hosts.

Finches
* Use Droncit™ as the main wormer.
* Use Coopex™ or Avian Insect Liquidator™ to help control tapeworm intermediate hosts.

Parrots and Pigeons
* Use Panacur 25™, Cydectin™ or Ivomec Liquid for Sheep™, Nilverm™ or Wormout™ gel by crop needle.
   or
* Use Panacur 25™ or Droncit™ mixed in with suitable favourite food.
   or
* Use Nilverm™, Wormout™ gel, Avitrol Plus™, Ivomec Liquid for Sheep™, Synanthic™, Systemex™ or Benzelmin™ in the drinking water or tablets in pigeons.
   or
* Use Ivomec Pour-on for Cattle™ as drops on the skin at the base of the neck.
   as well
* Use management to minimise the birds' contact with parasite eggs on the floor.

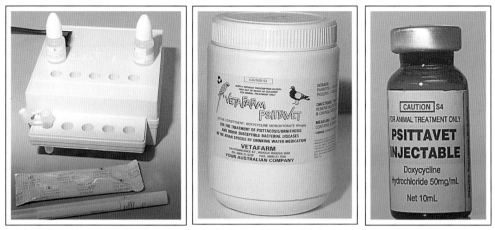

Left: The Clearview™ test used to detect Chlamydophila psittaci (Psittacosis) in sick birds. It is not as useful in birds that are not sick.
Centre: Psittavet™ – the powder form.
Right: Psittavet™ – the injectable form. One of the best antibiotics for Psittacosis.

PSITTACOSIS (Chlamydophilosis)

While this disease is mentioned in other places in this book, it is such an important disease and it is a danger to both you and your birds, that I felt we needed to emphasise it by allocating it a separate chapter.

The organism that causes Psittacosis was, until recently, called *Chlamydia psittaci*. The name has been changed to *Chlamydophila psittaci*. This is a bit of a tongue twister but as science advances, names are changed for reasons of accuracy. This organism has a wide host spectrum among birds, all the parrots and at least 130 non-parrot species, particularly pigeons. It also affects mammals (horses, cattle, sheep, roebuck, domesticated cats, guinea pigs, koalas, dogs and humans).

Chlamydophila psittaci can be highly contagious. It causes a disease called Psittacosis in parrots and Ornithosis (by legal definition) in all other animals and humans. Because the same agent is involved, the use of the term Chlamydophilosis to describe infections caused by this organism should be encouraged. Chlamydophilosis is a reportable disease in many countries.

The signs of Chlamydophilosis are so variable that it can normally be ruled out only with laboratory investigations. The more common rule-outs include infections with *Herpesvirus*, *Paramyxovirus*, Avian Influenza Virus Type A and *Enterobacteriaceae*, particularly Salmonellosis. The signs in the nervous system should be differentiated from Newcastle Disease and Salmonellosis, and the conjunctivitis in ducklings and goslings from Influenza A infections and Mycoplasmosis.

It is not uncommon for an apparently normal, healthy bird to be carrying Psittacosis in its system. It is possible for birds to remain this way for the whole of their life. On occasions they may shed the *Chlamydophila psittaci* in their droppings or secretions from their respiratory tract and pass the infection on to other birds or in-contact animals, including humans.

Psittacosis is a disease that commonly occurs in birds that have been stressed – in a shop, newly introduced to an aviary, in a moult, subject to overcrowding or bullying from other birds etc. **It is the most common cause of death in birds within two weeks of purchase.**

Diagnosis of Psittacosis

The signs are not specific and can mimic a large range of diseases. Therefore, tests and an examination by an experienced avian veterinarian are often essential to differentiate Psittacosis from other diseases. This is complicated by the fact that the *Chlamydophila psittaci* can lower the bird's immune system, making it more prone to developing secondary infection. This allows the *Chlamydophila psittaci* as well as another disease to be in the bird's system. The signs you see in the bird are caused by the secondary disease but underlying this problem, the actual cause is the *Chalmydophila psittaci*.

Birds with Psittacosis will not always look sick. They may just have poor breeding results, deaths in the nest and an occasional bird will die – this is the tip of the iceberg. A bird with Psittacosis can appear normal but then develop signs of illness when it is placed under some stress.

Clinical Examination
Any of the following signs alone or in any combination can be seen:
- Depression.
- Not eating.
- Weight loss.
- Watery eyes.
- Excess urine (often green).
- Diarrhoea (bright green to black).
- Runny nose.
- Blinking or partly closed eyes.
- Plugging of nostrils.
- Sneezing.

Clinical Pathology
These tests are used in the laboratory:
- Complement-fixation test (CFT).
- Immunofluorescence.
- DNA testing (eg polymerase chain reaction – PCR)
- ELISA (eg Clearview™ test).
- Isolation and growth of *Chlamydophila psittaci*.

Radiology
Splenic enlargement – not a specific but a suspicion.

Post-Mortem Examination
There is no single sign that will diagnose Psittacosis at post-mortem examination. Laboratory tests must be performed to confirm the diagnosis.

At post-mortem examination, the changes seen are quite variable and include:
- Thickened air sacs (they are normally thin and easy to see through).
- Swollen spleen (more commonly seen in parrots than pigeons).
- Swollen liver (edges are not sharp).
- Jelly-like clots throughout the air sacs and abdomen.
- Inflammation of the lungs, intestines and kidneys.

Important Facts about Psittacosis
- Surveys indicate that between 30% and 70% of the birds tested, mostly parrots, have anti-chlamydial antibodies. Clinical disease is precipitated mainly by human induced conditions and procedures.
- *Chlamydophila psittaci* can usually be detected in the faeces ten days prior to the onset of clinical signs.
- Carriers may begin to shed the organism following a stressful event or disease.
- Antibody production with an active infection may be poor, and birds that survive infection are fully susceptible to disease again soon after recovery.
- The most common cause of Air Sacculitis and Septicaemia in Australian parrots and

pigeons. Occasionally seen in Budgerigars and finches.

- Generally not as acute an onset as with bacterial Septicaemia. Associated with times of stress in an aviary.
- Very common in the *Neophema* genus (Bourke's, Scarlet-chested, Turquoise, Elegant, Blue-winged Parrots etc) and the *Polytelis* genus (Princess, Superb and Regent Parrots).
- Outbreaks begin in late summer, peak in autumn and remain high throughout winter.

Psittacosis in People

The most common way people can be infected is by inhaling aerosols from droppings, feather dust or respiratory tract excretions (particularly sneezing).

In people the incubation period is 4–15 days. Clinical signs usually have rapid onset and include headache, fever, irritant and non-productive cough, chills, loss of appetite, harsh breathing sounds, chest pains and generalised pains, lethargy and a sore throat. In many cases it is mistaken for a bout of influenza. In untreated cases, relapses are common. Reinfection is possible soon after recovery. Complications can include infections of the muscle or lining of the heart which can lead to death, particularly in the very young or the aged. Because *Chlamydophila psittaci* can suppress the immune system, secondary bacterial infections can occur. Psittacosis in most people is often only mild and is easily treated by your doctor. It is potentially a more serious prospect for anyone who is sick, elderly or immunosuppressed (eg AIDS or transplant patients). These people need to discuss this with their doctor.

Death can occur if the Psittacosis is left untreated. If you have any of the signs above mention to your doctor that you have regular contact with birds. The organism can be excreted in the sputum of infected humans as well as eye and nasal excretions. It can also be excreted in the faeces.

Chlamydophila psittaci is quite a strong organism and can survive well in the environment. It has been known to survive on glass or in straw for three weeks, in bird seed for two months, in poultry litter for up to eight months and in frozen turkey for longer than twelve months.

The most common source of *Chlamydophila psittaci* is airborne dried matter containing faeces, eye or nasal discharge, litter, feathers, straw/dust or dander.

The habit of kissing birds or any close proximity of your face to a bird is a potential for disease transmission and should be discouraged.

Treatment of Birds

In individual birds, the preferred treatment for Psittacosis is an antibiotic (Doxycycline™ or azithromycin) delivered via intramuscular injection or crop needle. Some birds, despite correct dosing will have relapses. This is because the *Chlamydophila psittaci* organisms survive deep within cells in the bird's bone marrow and medication does not penetrate well into this area. In extreme cases, intravenous injection may be preferred.

Where a large number of birds are involved, the only practical method of medicating is via the drinking water. Be aware that this method is unreliable because it requires the bird to drink sufficient quantities of medicated water at regular intervals or there will not be sufficient drug in the bird's system to effectively combat the disease.

All the drugs listed below are broken down by exposure to light and temperature. The in-water medication is best made fresh each day and replaced in the evening. With this, the birds take a good drink in the evening, the drug is exposed to minimal light and heat during the night so it is still potent in the morning when they again take a good drink. The medication will break down through the day and then be strong again when replaced in the evening. In this way the birds have the best chance of taking in an effective amount of the medication. All medicated water should be placed in a shaded spot in the aviary.

Suggested Medications and Treatments
Chlortetracycline (CTC) (Aureomycin™, Tricon™)
- **Dose:**
- ***Parrots:*** 500mg/L of water for 30 days quarantine period.
- ***Lorikeets:*** Use nectar formula with 0.05% CTC for 45 days.
- ***Flock:*** 150mg/L of water for 45 days.
- ***Individual:*** 10mg/60ml of mash. Force feed 20ml per 100 gram body weight every eight hours.

In all cases the CTC must be made freshly each day. Provide this medicated water/nectar only in glass, glazed earthenware or plastic containers, not metal (other than stainless steel). Remove all sources of calcium such as shellgrit or cuttlebone, as it strongly chelates (binds) the CTC. CTC can adversely affect fertility for 4–6 weeks.

or

Doxycycline (Psittavet™, Vibramycin™, Vibravet™)
- **Dose:**
- 25–50mg/kg every 24 hours orally for 45 days.
- 10g/L in-water medication for 45 days.
- 75–100mg/kg every 7 days by intramuscular injection x 6–8 injections. (75mg/kg for conures, macaws and lovebirds; 100mg/kg for all other parrots).

The only safe forms for intramuscular injection are:
Vibravenos SF™ 20mg/ml (Pfizer).
- **Dose:**
- 0.35–0.5ml per 100 gram body weight once weekly for 6–8 weeks.

or

Psittavet™ **injectable** 50mg/ml (Vetafarm).
- **Dose:**

  Manufacturer recommends using 0.1ml per 100 gram body weight once weekly for 6–7 weeks.

  All other injectable forms must be given intravenously.

or

Enrofloxacin™ (Baytril).

  15–30mg/kg twice daily for 14 days orally or by intramuscular injection.

During Treatment Period
- Minimise stress.
- Cease breeding.
- Do not introduce new birds.
- Remove any bullies.
- Improve diet.
- Provide a secure aviary.
- Provide protection from the elements.
- Clean and disinfect the aviary approximately every two weeks during treatment. Wear a face mask when cleaning. Dilute all your disinfectants exactly according to the manufacturer's directions.
- Allow two to four weeks after treatment before commencing breeding.

DISINFECTION

There is no disinfectant that is suitable for all occasions. You need to evaluate your situation and then choose carefully.

In all cases, the disinfectant must be used strictly according to the manufacturer's instructions. The commonly thought principle that 'using it at a stronger concentration so it will be more effective' is both dangerous to your birds and incorrect. Most disinfectants are actually less effective at stronger concentrations.

The build-up of most infectious agents can be controlled simply by washing with hot water and a good detergent. The aim is to have the surface visibly clean. Disinfectants should only be used when you need them – when there is a disease outbreak.

Nearly all disinfectants are inactivated when any organic material is present. For the disinfectant to work properly you need the area to be visibly clean. Any organic material or debris must be thoroughly removed – you need to remove all feathers including dust and dander, any droppings or other body excretions and any food material. Putting a disinfectant on top of any of this material means that you have wasted your time and effort. There is an old saying, that 'disinfection is 99% elbow grease and 1% chemicals'.

Any disinfectant solution must be in contact with the area being disinfected for 15 to 30 minutes to be effective. Once this time has passed, the area must be thoroughly rinsed to remove any residue that may harm the birds. You must never return birds to an area that has not been thoroughly rinsed.

All disinfectants should be stored in a closed cupboard in an area away from the birds or their food.

Take care using disinfectants around hatchlings and other young birds as they are more likely to have problems with fumes from disinfectants compared to larger birds. Make sure airflows in nurseries are high enough to remove all fumes.

How do you know which product is actually in the bottle in your hand? By law, all products must have the active constituent or ingredient listed prominently on the label. Read the label and then find the active constituent. Identify it in the list following. See if it is suitable for your needs.

Chlorhexidine

This product is gentle to body tissues – both human and birds. It is good for controlling viruses and Candidiasis (Thrush). It is not effective for many bacteria (especially Gram positive or *Pseudomonas*) or Psittacosis (*Chlamydophila psittaci*). In the correct dilution it is very useful to rinse or flush dirty wounds.

Common brand names are Aviclens™, Hibiclens™, Hibitane™ and Nolvosan™.

Quaternary Ammonium Compounds

This is a group of disinfectants. Sometimes they are called 'Quats'. Many of the disinfectants available in your supermarket contain these compounds. Those designed for use around the house are quite dilute but industrial strength is usually very concentrated. Follow all the manufacturer's instructions carefully.

These products are quite irritant to the skin. In high concentrations they can paralyse the bird's breathing. Used correctly they are extremely useful. They are very effective for *Chlamydophila* (Psittacosis) and many bacteria and viruses. Common situations where they are recommended are for washing down tables or soaking nets, dishes or perches.

Chlorine

This product bleaches and deodorises as well as killing many infectious agents. Be careful using it around any coloured fabrics as it will bleach and stain them. It breaks down quickly in bright light, especially sunlight. Any organic debris will inactivate it quickly. In high concentrations it is very irritant to the eyes, mouth and skin. It is not recommended for metal surfaces or equipment as it is quite corrosive. Avoid using the granulated form around birds, as it releases a heavy amount of fumes. Safer forms are household bleaches. Most bleaches are used at 200ml of bleach per 4 litres of water – but read the label to check this is correct.

A very useful form around many animals is chloramine. It combines chlorine and ammonia so that a lower dose of each is used. A common brand is Halamid™ or Halasept™.

Sodium hypochlorite is another common form of chlorine. The recommended strength to use this is at a 5% dilution. It is a very safe and effective agent. It is also the active constituent in many baby bottle sanitisers. Chlorine is very effective against the active, growing forms of viruses, bacteria, fungi and algae. It is not effective for their spores.

Tertiary Amines

These are relatively new disinfectants that are quite effective against a wide range of bacteria and viruses. In the diluted form they are safe around birds. They are quite useful for sterilising utensils and equipment used when handrearing birds. A common brand available is Avi-Safe™.

Iodine

Normal iodines are not used because they stain most surfaces. The best ones to use are the 'tamed iodines' – the iodophors. This has a slow release of iodine when used in its diluted form. They are not corrosive and only lightly staining – that washes out in water. They are very effective against a wide range of bacteria and fungi. They are not useful for viruses.

Common brands are Betadine™, Iovone™.

Glutaraldehyde

This is a very effective disinfectant that has a wide range of activity. It kills most bacteria, *Chlamydophila psittaci*, oocysts (Coccidiosis), and viruses. In the concentrated form it is extremely irritating to skin, eyes and mouth.

The major drawback is that it has been proven to cause cancer in humans with chronic exposure, so it must be used with protective clothing, boots etc. Common brands are Neo-Quat L.A.™ and Parvocide™.

Phenolics

These are a very early form of disinfectants. They include groups such as phenols, cresols and biphenyls. They have been used safely in the poultry industry for many years. OPP* is one of the newer and safer forms available. It is useful for many bacteria, fungi (including *Candida*) and viruses. It is not effective for *Chlamydophila psittaci* (Psittacosis). It is resistant to the presence of organic material and can be used for disinfecting of organic matter or for areas that are difficult to clean effectively.

The phenolics can be very irritant and are poisonous if eaten by the birds. Rinsing, after they are used, needs to be thorough. This is the form of disinfectant recommended by many government departments for quarantine applications.

*OPP is Sodium-O-phenylphenol. It is a relatively new form of phenolic disinfectant that is becoming more in favour around birds because it is less toxic than many of the older phenolics. It is commonly used in household and industrial disinfectants.

Alcohols

These are not commonly used for birds but may be used for some surfaces or instruments. They can be poisonous in concentrated forms and are irritant to most body tissues. They will help control many bacteria and some viruses. The most common

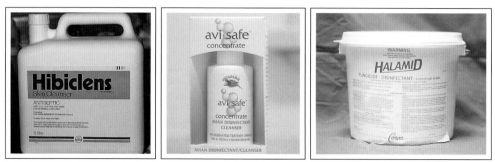

Left: Hibiclens™, a very useful disinfectant. Centre: Avi-safe™, a new and useful disinfectant. Right: Halamid™, also a useful disinfectant.

forms used are methylated spirits or isopropyl alcohol. These are available under many brand names.

Simple Disinfection Protocol

For food and water dishes, feeding devices as well as perches and accessories used in the aviary, use the following series of steps:

1. Soak for 30 minutes in either a phenolic or quaternary ammonium compound.
2. Place in a dishwasher on the hot water cycle.
3. Rinse thoroughly and dry.
4. Store in a closed, vermin-proof cupboard until used.

For cleaning your hands prior to and after handling birds, especially handrearing or ill birds, use an iodophor or chlorhexidine wash. Scrub your hands for at least five minutes. Most hand disinfectants need 5–10 minutes of contact to effectively clean your hands.

CONCLUSION

The purpose of this book is to provide the responsible aviculturist with the necessary information to be able to recognise, evaluate and respond to common diseases and ailments that affect captive held cage and aviary birds. However, it must be reiterated that your avian veterinarian is ultimately your best medium to maintain and treat a sick bird. With the information that can be gleaned from this book, and in conjunction with advice and guidance from your avian veterinarian, you will ensure that the health and condition of your birds and the management regime of your aviaries, will be the very best that you can provide.

FEATURES OF A TYPICAL BIRD

Crest
Orbital Ring
Crown
Forehead
Hindneck
Cere
Cheek
Bill
Neck
Chin
Mantle
Throat
Shoulder
Back
Breast
Wing Coverts
Rump
Secondary Feathers
Primary Feathers
Belly
Tail
Vent
Undertail
Abdomen

SKETCH BY RUSSELL KINGSTON

THE ALIMENTARY CANAL
OF A TYPICAL BIRD

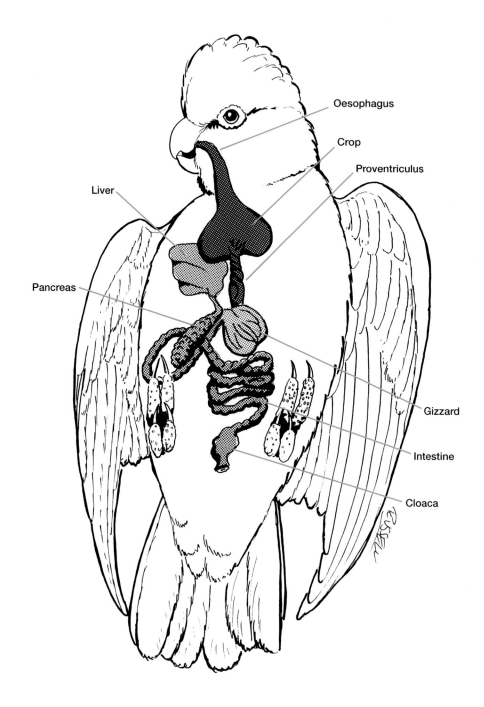

Oesophagus

Crop

Proventriculus

Liver

Pancreas

Gizzard

Intestine

Cloaca

SKETCH BY RUSSELL KINGSTON

THE RESPIRATORY TRACT OF A TYPICAL BIRD

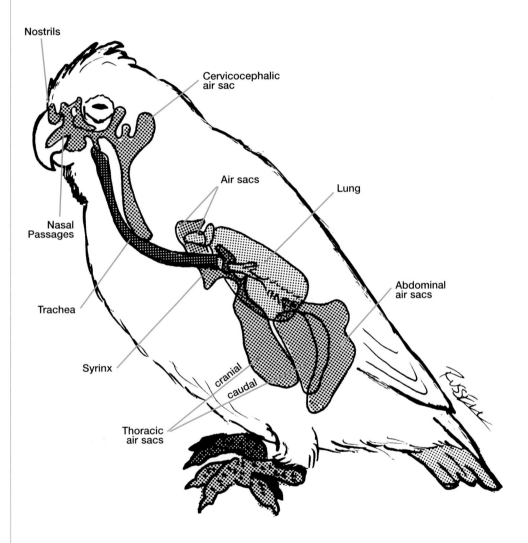

Nostrils

Cervicocephalic air sac

Air sacs

Lung

Nasal Passages

Abdominal air sacs

Trachea

Syrinx

cranial

caudal

Thoracic air sacs

SKETCH BY RUSSELL KINGSTON

TABLE OF ANTIBIOTICS

Many of the doses recommended today are based upon what has worked in the past. There is research being done at the moment to establish more specific dosages. Birds generally need higher doses than mammals. There is a large variation in the ability of different species of birds to absorb, use and excrete the same antibiotic. Eventually there will be doses recommended for each species. A lower dose is needed if given by injection compared to administering in-food or in-water.

ANTIBIOTIC	DURATION	BRAND NAMES	COMMENTS
Penicillins	5–10 days	Amoxil, Clavulox Penbritin, Orbenin	A lot of bacterial resistance in some instances. Very safe for the patient. Good for cat bite wounds. No allergy in birds.
		Piperacillin	Better for Gram negative than other Penicillins. Can only be given by injection.
Tetracyclines	30–45 days	Terramycin, Aureomycin Tricon, Panmycin Kanatet, Oxytetracycline Chlortetracycline Minocycline, Minomycin	Most commonly used for Psittacosis and Mycoplasmosis. Not very useful for intestinal infections. You must remove all sources of calcium from aviary eg cuttlefish, shellgrit, eggshells.
		Doxycycline Vibramycin, Doryc Psittavet, Vibravet	Best tetracycline drug for Psittacosis. Not affected by calcium as much. More useful for Gram negative infections than other tetracyclines.
Chloramphenicol	5–10 days	Chloromycetin Biomycetin	Unreliable absorption from the intestines. Best given by injection. Can be toxic for people with even minimal contact.
Erythromycin	10 days on 5 days off 10 days on	Gallimycin	Main use is for chronic respiratory disease, air sacculitis, mild sinusitis particularly if Mycoplasma is suspected. Most of the important bacteria are resistant to this.
Tylosin	10 days on 5 days off 10 days on	Tylan	Good for *Mycoplasma* infections, especially one-eyed cold. Can be bitter. Many bacteria are resistant.
Nitrofurans	7–10 days	Furadantin, Furoxone Furacin, Furasol, Neftin Furaltadone	Effective for bacteria in the bowel and some respiratory infections. Do not use with kidney disease. Can be toxic if overdosed. Use half dose in lorikeets and finches. Harmful to people, so most have been removed from sale.
Imidazoles	5–7 days	Emtryl	Emtryl can cause temporary infertility approx. 6 weeks. Easy to overdose – take care in hot weather and don't give to breeding birds or if feeding young as they drink a lot of water.
		Metrin, Flagyl, Torgyl Ronivet-S, Spartrix Turbosol	These are the safer forms, less likely to overdose.
Azithromycin	45 days	Zithromax	Has been used 1–2 times weekly for Psittacosis. It is being evaluated as a replacement for Doxycycline to treat *Chlamydophila psittaci*.

ANTIBIOTIC	DURATION	BRAND NAMES	COMMENTS
Aminoglycosides	5–10 days	Gentamicin, Gentam Garamycin, Gentocin	Not absorbed from the intestines, so you need to give by injection. Can be toxic especially to kidneys. Active against many Gram negative bacteria.
		Amikacin, Amiglyde-V	Same as Gentamicin but less toxic. Give with plenty of fluids. Best aminoglycoside for birds.
Linocomycin	5–10 days	Lincocin	Not very effective in birds except in some skin infections.
Lincomycin & Spectinomycin	2–4 weeks	Lincospectin	There is a high level of resistance in Australia. May need to add sweetener. Injectable form useful for respiratory disease in parrots, especially Eclectus.
Sulphonamides	5–10 days	Dimivec, Embazin Gantrasin, Salazopyrin Vetisulid	Can have high levels of resistance. Useful for some respiratory infections and Coccidiosis. High doses can damage the kidneys especially in dehydrated birds.
Sulphonamides Trimethoprim	5–10 days	Tribrissen, Trivetrin Trimsul	Less resistance than sulphonamides alone. Used for intestinal infections such as *Coccidia, E. coli* and other Gram negative infections especially in nestlings. High doses can damage the kidneys especially in dehydrated birds. May cause some birds to vomit.
Quinolones	Up to 2 weeks	Enrofloxacin, Ciprofloxacin Baytril, Cartril	Use with care in juvenile birds, may cause joint damage. Excellent action against Mycoplasma, most Gram negative and many Gram positive bacteria as well as *Chlamydophila*. Available as water soluble liquid and injection.
Cephalosporins *First generation*	5–10 days	Celphalexin, Cephalothin	Active against most Gram positive and some Gram negative bacteria.
Second generation	5–10 days	Cefoxitin	More active against Gram negative bacteria. Injectable form only.
Third generation	5–10 days	Cefotaxime, Ceftriaxone	Active against most Gram negative including *Pseudomonas*. Cephalosporins not as commonly used in Australia as the USA.
Toltrazuril	3 days	Baycox, Carlox	Most effective drug currently available for Coccidiosis.
Nystatin	5–10 days	Mycostatin, Nilstat	Useful for infections in mouth crop or intestines caused by yeasts, especially *Candida* in handreared juveniles.

COMMON PARASITICIDES

These are what are commonly used. Be aware that they are usually not registered for use in this manner or in the species you are treating. For this reason the doses and recommendations in this section are subject to the consideration that all persons using these drugs do so entirely at their own risk.

DRUG	BRAND (TM)	STRENGTH	DIRECTIONS
Levamisole	L-Spartakon Tablets	20mg	Use 1 tablet per 500 gram bird.
	Nilverm Pig & Poultry Wormer	16mg/ml	Finches: Use 40ml per litre water for 24 hours. Parrot Finches: Use a half dose (20ml per litre water). Repeat one day a week for a total of four weeks. Parrots: Use 50ml per litre of water for 24 hours.
	Nilverm Oral Drench	32mg/ml	Use 25ml per litre of water.
	Nilverm Oral LV	80mg/ml	Mix with water in a 1:1 ratio and give 0.1ml per 100 gram body weight by crop needle for 3 consecutive days. In-water: Use 9ml per litre of water.
	Nilverm Injection	89mg/ml	Use 8ml per litre of water.
	Avitrol Syrup	Levamisole 10mg/ml	Finches: Use 1 drop per 15 gram and 3 drops per 30 gram body weight. Budgerigar: Use 5 drops per 50 gram body weight. Cockatiel: Use 8 drops per 80 gram body weight. Cockatoo: Use 50 drops per 500 gram body weight.
	Vital Tablets	20mg	Use 1 tablet per 500 gram body weight.
Oxfendazole	Synanthic	18.12g/L	Finches: Use 25ml per litre of water for 3 days. Parrots: Dilute 1ml per 3ml of water and give 0.25ml per 100 gram body weight by crop needle for 3-5 days.
	Systamex	90.6g/L	Finches: Use 5ml per litre of water for 3 days. Parrots: Dilute 1ml with 20ml of water and give 0.25ml per 100 gram body weight by crop needle for 3-5 days.
	Benzelmin	200g/L	Finches: Use 2.2ml per litre of water for 3 days. Parrots: Dilute 1ml with 50ml water and then give 0.25ml per 100 gram body weight by crop needle for 3-5 days.
Fenbendazole	Panacur 25	25mg/ml	Use 8ml per kg of soaked seed for 5 days. Gavage/oral use 0.1-2ml per 50 gram body weight for 3 days consecutively. Nectar mix: Use 8ml per litre of nectar.
	Panacur 100	100mg/ml	Not recommended even if diluted to above dose. Fatalities have been recorded with this preparation.
Albendazole	Valbazen	113mg/ml	Finches: 5ml per litre of water for 3 days. Make fresh each 24 hours. Offer clear water for 2 days then repeat. Direct to the beak: 0.05ml per 100 gram body weight once daily for 3 days or 0.1ml per 100 gram body weight as a single dose.
Ivermectin	Ivomec Liquid for Sheep	0.8g/L	0.1ml of this product per 100 gram body weight into the beak. No dilution is required for parrots and pigeons.
	Ivomec Pour-on for Cattle	5.0g/L	Apply 0.015ml per 100 gram body weight placed on skin at back of the neck. Alternatively dilute 1ml with 9ml of propylene glycol and use 0.15ml per 100 gram body weight. This product is suitable for penetrating the skin.

DRUG	BRAND (TM)	STRENGTH	DIRECTIONS
Ivermectin	Ivomec Antiparasitic injection for cattle	10g/L	Parrots: Dilute 1ml with 100ml propylene glycol. Give 0.2ml per 100 gram body weight by crop needle.
	Ivomec RV for Sheep	2g/L	Dilute with water immediately before use. Mix 1ml with 1.0ml of water. Use 0.1ml of this mix per 100 gram body weight by crop needle.
Moxidectin	Cydectin	100 mcg/ml	Aviary birds in-water dose: 20ml per litre of drinking water. Pigeons: Individual adult bird dose: 0.25ml into the mouth or crop. Flock dose: 5ml per litre of water for 24 hours. Finches: Individual dose: 0.1ml per 50 gram body weight into the crop. Flock dose: 5ml per litre of water for 3-5 days, made fresh daily.
Praziquantel	Droncit	Cat tablet 23mg Dog tablet 50mg	Finches: Use 50mg per kg of seed. Crush the tablet and mix with a small amount of vegetable oil or cod liver oil. Mix through the seed. Feed fresh each day for 3 days. Repeat dose in 10-14 days. Parrots: Crush 1 Droncit cat tablet (23mg) or 1/2 Droncit dog tablet (50mg) and mix with 1.0ml water in a syringe. Give 0.1ml per 100 gram body weight, immediately the solution is mixed, before it begins to settle out.
	Prazivet Solution	25mg/ml	Mix 5ml per litre of drinking water. Leave in the aviary for 24 hours then replace with fresh water.
Toltazuril	Baycox	25g/L	Most birds: 3ml per litre of drinking water for 3 days. Pigeons: 2ml per litre of drinking water for 2 days. Budgerigars: 3ml per litre of drinking water for 2-5 days.
Amprolium	Amprolmix Plus	Amprolium 250g/kg + Ethopabate 16g/kg	Week 1: 3ml per litre of water. Week 2: 2ml per litre of water. Week 3: 1ml per litre of water. Then 1ml per litre of water for 1 week each month.
	Coccivet	Amprolium 80g/L + Ethopabate 5.1g/L	Use 1.5ml per litre of drinking water for 5-7 days.
	Amprolium 200		Follow manufacturer's directions.
Permethrin	Avian Insect Liquidator		For parrots, finches and canaries use a 5% solution. Mix 1 part concentrate made up to 20 parts total volume with water (add 1ml to 19ml water). Place solution in a spray pump. Hold the spray 30-40cm from the birds and apply 4-5 sprays (3-4ml) to the bird. Also spray cages, aviaries, perches and nestboxes thoroughly with the diluted product. Repeat every 6 weeks or as required.

DRUG COMBINATIONS

DRUG	BRAND (TM)	STRENGTH	DIRECTIONS
Levamisole & Praziquantel	Avitrol Plus Syrup	Levamisole 10mg/ml + Praziquantel 2mg/ml	Give 1 drop per 10 gram body weight into the beak or 1ml per 20ml of drinking water for 24 hours.
	Avitrol Plus Tablet	Levamisole 20mg + Praziquantel 4mg	Use 1/2 a tablet for 250-500 gram bodyweight. Use 1 tablet for 500-750 gram body weight.
Oxfendazole & Praziquantel	Wormout Tablets	Oxfendazole 20mg + Praziquantel 20mg	Give 1 tablet per 2kg body weight.
	Wormout Gel	Oxfendazole 20g/L + Praziquantel 20g/L	Use 1ml per 80ml of drinking water. Supply for 2 days, individual bird dose is 0.05ml per 100 gram body weight as a single dose. Repeat every 3 months.

The Acclaimed 'A Guide to ...' range

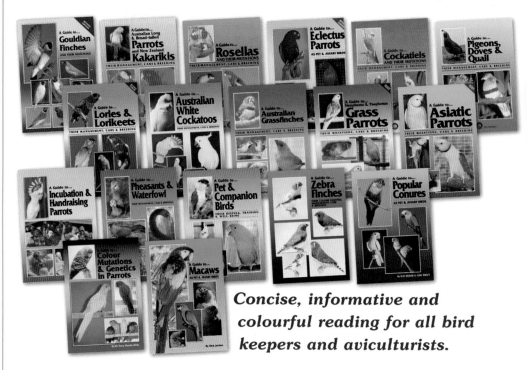

Concise, informative and colourful reading for all bird keepers and aviculturists.

- A Guide to Gouldian Finches (Revised Edition)
- A Guide to Australian Long and Broad-tailed Parrots and New Zealand Kakarikis
- A Guide to Rosellas and Their Mutations
- A Guide to Eclectus Parrots (Revised Edition)
- A Guide to Cockatiels and Their Mutations
- A Guide to Pigeons, Doves and Quail
- A Guide to Lories and Lorikeets (Revised Edition)
- A Guide to Australian White Cockatoos
- A Guide to Australian Grassfinches
- A Guide to Neophema and Psephotus Grass Parrots and Their Mutations (Revised Edition)
- A Guide to Asiatic Parrots and Their Mutations (Revised Edition)
- A Guide to Incubation and Handraising Parrots
- A Guide to Pheasants and Waterfowl
- A Guide to Pet and Companion Birds
- A Guide to Zebra Finches
- A Guide to Popular Conures as Pet and Aviary Birds
- A Guide to Colour Mutations and Genetics in Parrots
- A Guide to Macaws as Pet and Aviary Birds
- Under the Microscope—Microscope Use and Pathogen Identification in Birds and Reptiles
- Handbook of Birds, Cages & Aviaries

ABK Publications stock a complete and ever increasing range of books and videos on all cage and aviary birds. For Free Catalogue and Price List see details opposite.

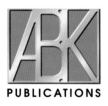

PUBLICATIONS